EBOLA

An In-Depth Insight for Nurses and Medical Professionals

by

Brenda L. Horsley RN

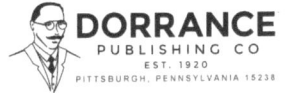

DORRANCE
PUBLISHING CO
EST. 1920
PITTSBURGH, PENNSYLVANIA 15238

Dorrance Publishing Co
585 Alpha Drive
Pittsburgh, PA 15238
Visit our website at www.dorrancebookstore.com

ISBN: 979-8-8860-4350-1
eISBN: 979-8-8860-4446-1

CONTENTS

INTRODUCTION TO EBOLA

With advancements in technology and research, the need for addressing and analyzing the causes and solutions to deadly diseases globally has gained momentum. It is not a newfound phenomenon that most illnesses and diseases have been around for a while now. They have picked up the pace, evolved, and morphed into new versions and mutations—each type deadlier than the previous one. Thus, finding a sustainable solution to these unwanted illnesses that have plagued societies has been a top priority worldwide.

One such disease in this regard is Ebola. Contrary to popular belief, this disease has been lingering across the continent of Africa for decades. Originating from the Democratic Republic of Congo, to quickly spreading like fire in Nigeria, Guinea, Sierra Leone, and even Liberia, this disease has managed to find a foothold everywhere. A few cases have even been reported in the Philippines, however, the only victims here have been animals.

The causes of Ebola have been linked to fruit bats. Labeled as a zoonotic disease, the primary host being a possible carrier can transmit the disease to a secondary host. These hosts such as chimpanzees, pigs, or gorillas can then infect a human. Being infected with Ebola thus becomes a source of concern.

The common reason being that the virus can be easily transferred to another human via the exchange of blood, bodily fluids, secretions, or organs. Even contact with an Ebola patient's mucus, bedding, or medical equipment can become deadly in this regard. So much so, that even unhealed, wounded, or broken skin can become a source of transmission.

With an outbreak having an intensity level such as this and occurring in sporadic intervals, a lot of investments in research and development have been undertaken. Safety protocols, along with treatment options and containment policy options have been observed, identified, and analyzed upon. Thus, the purpose of this course is to shed light on the characteristics, features, and sustainable policies at play in order to disseminate precise and accurate information to nurses, medical and environmental professionals.

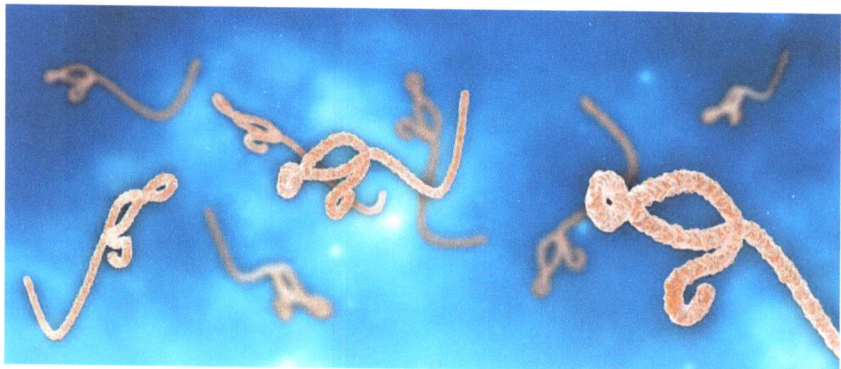

Figure 1. Ebola Virus Strain

THE HISTORY

To understand the contours of this disease, it is important to deconstruct its history and origin. By doing so a holistic picture can be created, taking all the key factors into perspective. Thus, ensuring robust and dynamic solutions going forward.

First discovered in 1976 in a small isolated village of Boende, Equateur, Ebola established its foothold in the Democratic Republic of Congo. The name comes from the Ebola River near the village where it took inception. Since then it has emerged and submerged in sporadic outbursts. What's more interesting is how it has evolved to different types over the years. Labeled as the Ebola Virus Disease (EVD) and Ebola Hemorrhagic Fever (RHF), this disease has crumbled and overwhelmed the already weak healthcare systems in many African countries.

From the remote areas of Central and West Africa, Ebola has taken the lives of many. Be it Guinea, Nigeria, Sierra Leone, and Liberia, it has infected thousands residing in these areas. And, the number of cases keeps growing with time. The reason being an institutional and structural weakness in the political-economic and social fabric of these countries. Engulfed with internal conflict and recovering from instability, these countries struggle with Ebola outbreaks when they occur. Everyone has been at-risk—nurses, healthcare workers, and doctors too. Experts such as, Sheik Umar Khan, Sierra Leones Ebola expert, and only virologist too succumbed to the Ebola virus in 2014.

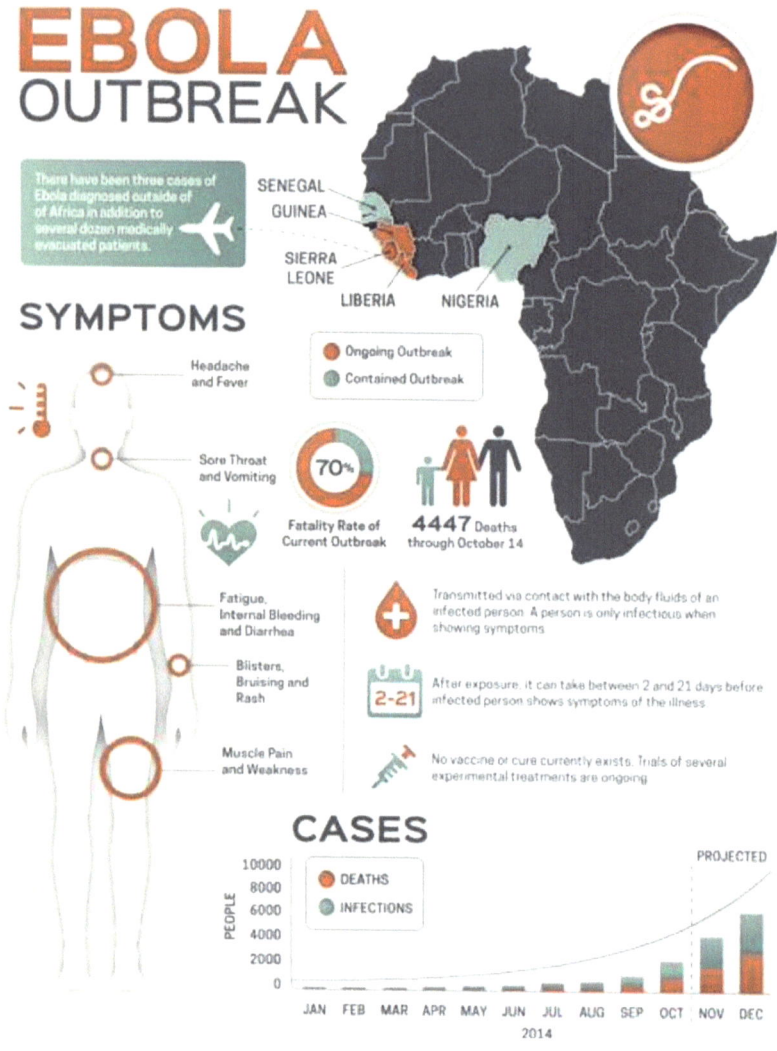

Figure 2 Ebola Outbreak in Africa - A Map

It is worth noting that Ebola outbreaks have not been confined to Africa. Cases have appeared in other countries worldwide. Spain for instance has had one reported case. Similarly, the United States has had two imported cases and two locally transmitted cases. They have been of five healthcare workers and one journalist, all of whom were transferred back home. The death of one of these healthcare workers, who was diagnosed with Ebola from Sierra Leone, took place on 17th November 2014, in Nebraska Medical Center. The Philippines has also confirmed cases of Ebola, however, they have been confined to animals only.

The table below is an overview of the previous Ebola outbreaks in chronological order. Highlighting the number of cases, deaths, and fatality percentage.

Table 1: Ebola virus outbreaks

Country	Cases	Deaths	Species	Year
Guinea	23	12	Zaire ebolavirus	2021
Dem. Rep of the Congo	12	6	Zaire ebolavirus	2021
Dem. Rep. of the Congo	130	55	Zaire ebolavirus	2020
Dem. Rep. of the Congo, Uganda	3470	2287	Zaire ebolavirus	2018-2020
Dem. Rep. of the Congo	54	33	Zaire ebolavirus	2018
Dem. Rep. of the Congo	8	4	Zaire ebolavirus	2017
Dem. Rep. of the Congo	66	49	Zaire ebolavirus	2014
Multiple countries	28646	11323	Zaire ebolavirus	2014-2016
Uganda	6*	3*	Sudan ebolavirus	2012
Dem. Rep. of the Congo	36*	13*	Bundibugyo ebolavirus	2012
Uganda	11*	4*	Sudan ebolavirus	2012
Uganda	1	1	Sudan ebolavirus	2011
Dem. Rep. of the Congo	32	15	Zaire ebolavirus	2008
Uganda	149	37	Bundibugyo ebolavirus	2007
Dem. Rep. of the Congo	264	187	Zaire ebolavirus	2007
Sudan (present day South Sudan)	17	7	Sudan ebolavirus	2004
Republic of Congo	35	29	Zaire ebolavirus	2003
Republic of Congo	143	128	Zaire ebolavirus	2002

Country	Cases	Deaths	Species	Year
Republic of Congo	57	43	*Zaire ebolavirus*	2001
Gabon	65	53	*Zaire ebolavirus*	2001
Uganda	425	224	*Sudan ebolavirus*	2000
South Africa	2	1	*Zaire ebolavirus*	1996
Gabon	60	45	*Zaire ebolavirus*	1996
Gabon	37	21	*Zaire ebolavirus*	1996
Zaire (present day DRC)	315	250	*Zaire ebolavirus*	1995
Côte d'Ivoire (Ivory Coast)	1	0	*Taï Forest ebolavirus*	1994
Gabon	52	31	*Zaire ebolavirus*	1994
Sudan (present day South Sudan)	34	22	*Sudan ebolavirus*	1979
Zaire (present day DRC)	1	1	*Zaire ebolavirus*	1977
Sudan (present day South Sudan)	284	151	*Sudan ebolavirus*	1976
Zaire (present day DRC)	318	280	*Zaire ebolavirus*	1976

Source: (Ebola Virus Disease Distribution Map: Cases of Ebola Virus Disease in Africa Since 1976, n.d.)

Source: (Ebola Virus Disease Distribution Map: Cases of Ebola Virus Disease in Africa Since 1976, n.d.)

The Origin in Question

It is widely believed that the Ebola virus could have originated from infected fruit bats. Thus confirming the Ebola virus as a zoonotic disease. It may transfer to a human being directly or via a host species such as infected primates, forest antelopes, or even pigs. Chimpanzees, gorillas, and apes are the primary host species for the Ebola virus. Fruit bats are a petri dish of bacteria and viruses, and their ability to fly makes it even easier for the transmission and spread of potential diseases.

In addition, it is interesting to note that the first-ever reported case of the Ebola virus was of a two-year-old boy and not an adult as generally assumed. After a lot of research, it has been deduced that other species of bats may have aided in the emergence of this disease. For instance, large colonies of free-tailed insectivorous bats reside in hollow trees. These areas are often places where village children gather around to play. Hence, making direct transmission possible.

Since then, five types of Ebola have been identified. This means that they are sub-types of the six species known today. These types are the Ebola-Zaire, Ebola-Sudan, Ebola-Bundibugyo, Tai Forest Ebola, and Ebola-Reston. From these, the deadliest have been the Bundibugyo Ebola virus, Sudan Ebola virus, and Zaire Ebola virus. The Zaire Ebola virus has given rise to the largest outbreak that is not just complicated in its nature but has been the most difficult one to contain as well. In 2014 it spread from a remote area in Southeast Guinea called Nzerekore to developed and urbanized areas within, including the capital of Guinea, Conakry.

A BREAKDOWN OF THE DISEASE

An insight into the devastating physical impacts of the Ebola virus has been known to all. Its lingering presence has been brought to light, observed, studied, and analyzed. The symptoms, diagnoses, and treatment options have evolved over the years. The different types have also been identified aiding towards the new and complicated developments at hand.

Taking its roots from the branch of Filoviruses, the Ebola virus is a subset of this family of viruses. The other two belonging to this family are the Cueva virus and the Marburg virus. Further, the Ebola virus has been demarcated into six species—four of which are known to impact the human body. That is, the Sudan virus, Ebola Zaire, Tai Forest, and the Bundibugyo virus. These species are named based on the location they originated from. In addition, each species comes with its types of the genus Ebolavirus.

The Leading Causes and Risks

Once transmitted via an infected bat and host species, the Ebola virus can quickly impact the human body. The transmission of the virus can find its way through many methods. The most common is the exchange of or coming in contact with infected bodily fluids. This also includes semen and urine. Ebola virus strains can be found in human semen for up to seven weeks even after having recovered.

Not just human contact, but the environment can also aid in the colonization of the virus. Contaminated medical equipment, clothing, and surfaces are labeled as primary carriers. While it is unclear for how long the virus may stay active on hard surfaces, experts believe it may be for up to six days. Thus frequent cleaning of surfaces with bleach or chlorine is recommended as it can kill the Ebola virus strains.

In addition, the incubation period of two days till twenty-one days has been ruled out as being confirmed. Confusions regarding whether the transmission rate is lower during cooler temperatures and the winter season are still unknown along with the cut back in the incubation timeline under such conditions.

We can discuss the dangers involved during funerals, then it's best to avoid direct contact with the body of the deceased. This is because the deceased person has a high viral load, making the virus easily transmissible to anyone that comes in contact with the body. Prior to death, bleeding is a common symptom. The infected blood thus is often carefully cleaned up and disposed of by trained Environmental Services Specialists (EVS).

In addition, many efforts have been made to create awareness and educate the masses on the risks. Medical charity organizations such as Medecins Sans Frontiers (MSF) have time and again disseminated information related to contracting the Ebola virus via touching the deceased loved one's body during religious worship and funeral services.

For grieving families, this situation is more difficult to deal with. This makes safe burial procedures complicated. However, there has been a shift and these procedures are now being encouraged by many. In places where outbreaks have been common, there has been a cultural shift towards understanding the risks and repercussions during burial, thus making the path towards creating more awareness easier.

More efforts are required to raise awareness about the devastating impacts of the Ebola virus on not just the patients infected, but the people around them and their loved ones. The ones in place have been promising and shown drastic improvements in recent years.

The Symptoms at Play

After the Ebola virus has been transmitted, the symptoms can begin to appear within two days. The incubation period of two to twenty-one days is the most crucial in this regard. However, the virus is only infectious once the symptoms begin to appear. These early signs are often common symptoms that come along with any other viral infection and thus make it easily transmissible during the initial stages.

The symptoms are sudden accompanied by the following characteristics.

EARLY SIGNS
High fever
Muscle pain
Anorexia
Headache
Chills
Weakness and fatigue
Joint pain

Once the first symptoms develop and progress, more severe symptoms may follow. These may include:

SERIOUS SYMPTOMS
Vomiting and stomach pain
Diarrhea
Skin irritation and rashes
Swollen genitals
Red eyes
Seizures
Internal and external bleeding in extreme cases. Bleeding of gums, the eyes, nose, ears, and rectum are common.
Low white blood cells and platelet counts – identified via blood tests
Dehydration and extreme loss of body fluids

Low blood pressure
Elevated liver and kidney enzymes along with similar symptoms of impaired liver and kidneys
Multiple organ failure – this can eventually lead to death

If any of the initial symptoms occur, the patient should isolate themselves and get in touch with the nearest medical expert or facility. Early diagnosis and treatment are key towards ensuring quick recovery from the Ebola virus and warranting its transmission are contained.

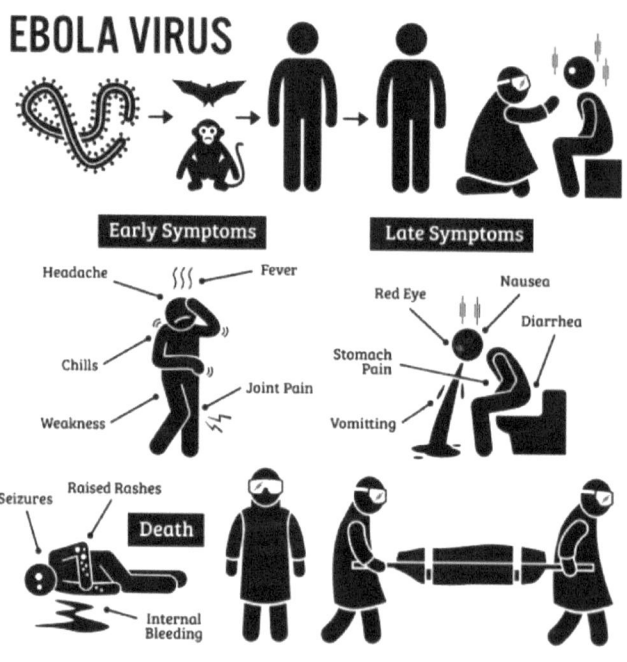

Figure 3 Ebola Virus Symptoms

The Diagnosis

Since the symptoms of the Ebola virus mimic that of Typhoid, Meningitis, and Malaria in its initial stages, diagnosis can be complicated. Here, a breakdown of the patient's medical history, work-life, travel experience, and contact with wildlife is taken into account. To rule out Ebola a series of blood tests are required. This is to be conducted urgently especially if the person suspected of having the Ebola virus has recently traveled to an area where there had been an Ebola virus outbreak or case.

Multiple blood tests can be administered to rule out the possibility of the Ebola Virus along with its specific type. The of the common ones are as follows:

- √ Serum Neutralization Test
- √ Antibody-Capture Enzyme-Linked Immunosorbent Assay (ELISA) – this is conducted for a real-time diagnosis
- √ Virus Isolation via the cell nature
- √ Antigen-capture detection tests
- √ Reverse Transcriptase Polymerase Chain Reaction (RT-PCR)
- √ Electron Microscopy – this can help identify filovirions in cell cultures due to their distinctive filamentous shapes

In addition, it is important to note that samples drawn from patients for diagnosis require careful handling, storage, and transportation. Maximum biological containment conditions are created for testing on non-inactivated samples to ensure the safety and protection of all stakeholders involved.

The Treatment Options & Complications
While the research on the Ebola virus has been ongoing for decades, there has been no FDA- approved vaccine or antiviral drug available yet. Vaccine trials are still underway and once approved and successful, healthcare workers will be ensured as the first receivers. As time progresses, it would soon be available to the masses, however for now the likelihood of this happening anytime soon seems meek.

In addition, many potential treatments have emerged in the pipeline as well. They involve immune therapies, drug therapies, and blood products from Ebola virus survivors. There are basic intervention methods and protocols that are followed by health care professionals to help patients recover. Some of these interventions are as follows.

√ Monitoring blood pressure

√ Ensuring the patient is well hydrated via intravenous fluids and electrolytes; oral fluids are also encouraged to revive body salts and ensure quick recovery

√ Maintaining and monitoring of oxygen levels

√ In extreme cases, blood transfusions may be needed

√ Treating and addressing infections as they appear

These recovery mechanisms depend on how adequate the supportive care is and how strong the immune system of the person infected is. After recovering from the Ebola virus, the patient has enough antibodies that can last for up to ten years, in some cases even longer than this. There is no guarantee that these survivors with antibodies will not be infected by different species of the Ebola virus.

Not only this, but many people that have recovered have developed long-term complications. Some of them include prolonged joint pain and vision problems.

The case of Richard Sara is particularly interesting. He was a doctor from Massachusetts who recovered from Ebola after being hospitalized for weeks. After recovering he was hospitalized once again due to a respiratory condition coupled with a pink eye unrelated to Ebola. This has brought to light the need for determining what factors allow some patients to recover while others are unable to.

ENSURING SAFETY FOR THE RELEVANT STAKEHOLDERS – NURSES, HEALTHCARE WORKERS, AND DOCTORS

Amidst concerning and stressful outbreaks, ensuring containment is important. There is another element that requires strong attention. And that is of ensuring safety for relevant healthcare team involved. While patients themselves are provided supportive basic intervention, nurses' and healthcare workers' safety is often overlooked. They are the ones at most risk due to their close proximity to Ebola patients. Despite having personal protective equipment and clothing such as full body suits, masks, and goggles, many nurses and healthcare workers have still been infected and succumbed to the disease. Due to this, there have been numerous demands by nurses for better protective equipment along with training procedures to ensure their safety and protection.

But first, to improve safety measures and ensure protection, it's best to identify which individuals fall under the umbrella of healthcare personnel (HCP). They are as follows:

- Management
- Physicians
- Nurses, and nursing assistants
- All persons working in health care facilities and settings that are prone to have exposure to Ebola patients or infected materials such as body substances, medicals supplies, aerosols, etc. This includes trained Environmental Services Specialists (EVS), supply chain, engineers, and respiratory therapists.
- Medical experts
- Therapists (respiratory and physical)

- Technicians and emergency medical staff at hospitals and clinics
- Pharmacists
- Laboratory and autopsy personnel/assistants
- Medical students and trainees
- Healthcare personnel at home
- Individuals not involved in patient care but at risk of exposure such as environmental services, security personnel, and volunteers

Health care personnel should therefore be provided with adequate training and guidelines related to taking care of Ebola patients. These need to be repeated in systematic intervals in order to ensure competency in Ebola-related infection control protocols. Donning (putting on of PPE) and Doffing (Removal of PPE) in this regard is a top priority. For this, a trained observer needs to be present at all times to ensure the proper procedure for donning and doffing is followed.

The recommended Personal Protective Equipment can be of two types. Either the PAPR (powered air-purifying respirators) or N95 Respirator.

The PAPR consists of a face shield that covered the entire face. It may be in the form of a helmet or headpiece. If using a reusable one, then this headpiece requires coverage with a single-use hood that is disposable. It usually extends to the shoulders and covers the neck entirely.

The N95 Respirator on the other hand is a single-use PPE with a disposable single hood that extends to the shoulders. It also includes a full face shield. However, it is required that healthcare workers do not inadvertently touch their faces under the face shield during patient care.

Donning and Doffing Procedures

These procedures require strict adherence to guidelines and protocols that have been kept in place.

Donning of PAPR/N95 Personal Protective Equipment

A designated place for doffing is essential to start off. The following is the breakdown of the process.

1. Trained Observers presence—the steps for Donning need to be read aloud by this supervisor to ensure proper donning of the PPE. The supervisor also confirms each step has been carried out properly and verifies to see that no part of the skin or hair is exposed at the end.

2. Removal of personal clothing and wearing of scrubs, disposable garments, and washable shoes. This also includes the removal of any jewelry, watches, cell phones, pens, etc.

3. Inspection of PPE to ensure it is the correct size and serviceable.

4. Hand hygiene followed by putting on inner gloves and shoe covers.

5. Wearing of the gown. Here tucking in the cuffs of the inner gloves under the sleeves of the gown are important. For PAPR with a self contained blower unit, this needs to be worn before wearing the gown. For the PAPR with an external belt-mounted blower, it is to be worn on top of the gown. In the case of an N95 PPE, wearing of the N95 respirator is carried out here ensuring a user seal check. This is followed by wearing the surgical hood ensuring coverage of the hair, ears, neck, and shoulders. The apron is also put on after this step.

6. Wearing outer gloves with cuffs pulled over the gown sleeves.

7. Putting on the respirator with the PAPR face shield or helmet. If the PAPR with a self-contained blower unit is integrated inside the helmet or the PAPR external belt-mounted blower unit with an attached re-

usable headpiece is used, then it should extend to the shoulders and cover the neck, including hair and ears. For the N95 PPE, the face shield is worn here.

8. Wearing of the outer apron for additional protection (For PAPR PPE).

9. Verification by the trained officer.

10. Disinfection of outer gloves before entering patient care area.

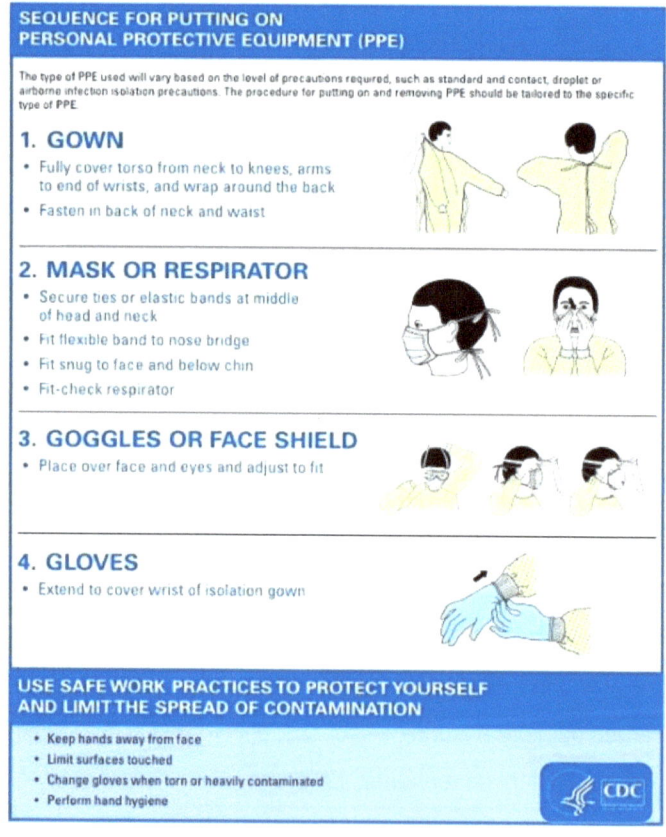

Figure 4 Sequence for Donning

Doffing of PAPR/N95 Personal Protective Equipment

The removal of PPE too needs to be carried out in a designated PPE removal area. All the items removed need to be contained in a leak-proof waste container.

Here is a breakdown of the donning process:

1. Trained Observers presence—the steps for Donning need to be read aloud by this supervisor to ensure proper removal of the PPE. Reminders of not touching the face or performing any other reflexive action are to be provided as well

2. Inspection of the PPE for any visible cuts, abrasions, or tears before removal. If contaminated, the PPE requires effective disinfection using an EPA registered disinfectant.

3. Disinfection of outer gloves.

4. Removal of apron by rolling it from the inside to the outside.

5. Inspection for any tears or contamination once again. If needed, disinfection is to be followed as done previously.

6. DIsinfection of outer gloves followed by removal of shoe covers.

7. Disinfection of outer gloves and removal

8. Inspection and Disinfection of inner gloves—check for any tears, cuts, or visible contamination and disinfect

9. Removal of inner gloves, perform hand hygiene and put on a clean pair of gloves

10. Removal of PAPR respirator components while disinfecting gloves at each step. Place reusable components in the area or container designated for disinfection.

   If wearing an N95 respirator, then removal of face shield while avoiding touching of the face. Similar is the protocol for removal of the surgical hood. Disinfection of inner gloves is followed in between each step here as well.

11. Removal of the gown while being careful of inner garments or scrubs coming in contact with the outer surface of the gown. Discard gown once removed.

12. Disinfection of inner gloves and washable shoes. Repetition of disinfection of inner gloves once again.

    For N95 PPE, removal and discarding of the respirator followed by disinfection of gloves is conducted.

13. Inspection of the healthcare worker for any contamination. If identified, an infection preventionist or safety and health coordinator must be informed immediately before exiting the PPE removal area

14. A shower followed by medical assessment and protocol evaluation by the infection preventionist or occupational safety and health coordinator.

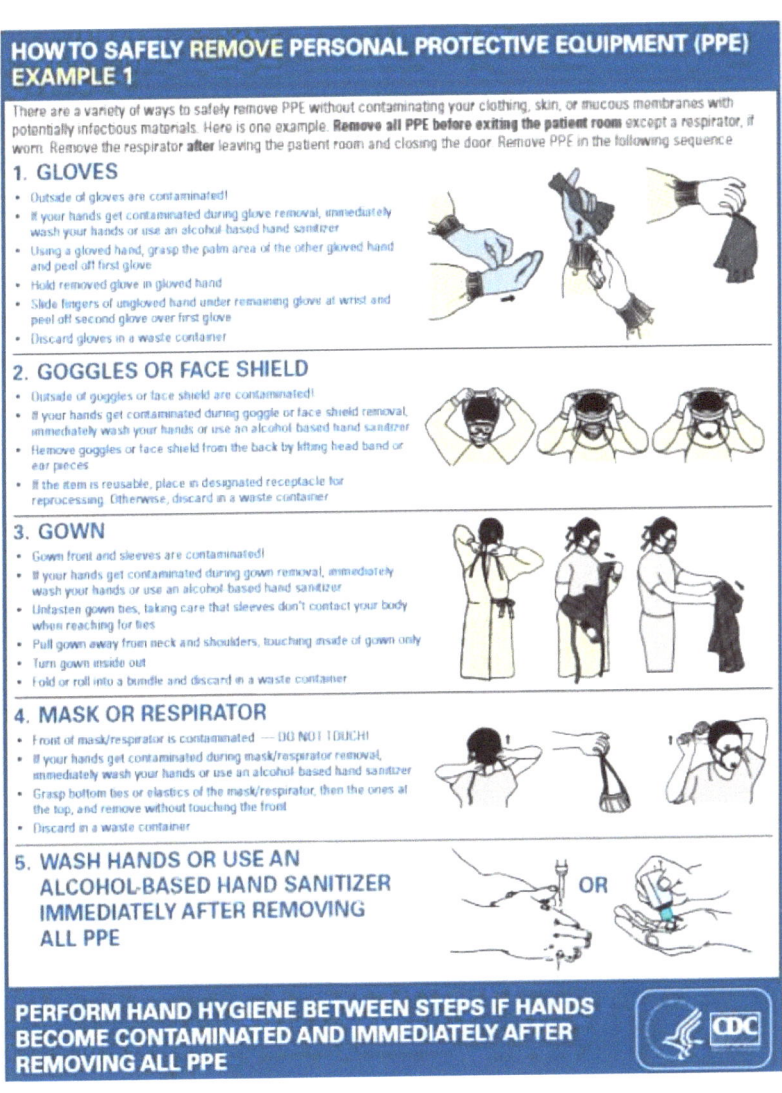

HOW TO SAFELY REMOVE PERSONAL PROTECTIVE EQUIPMENT (PPE) EXAMPLE 1

There are a variety of ways to safely remove PPE without contaminating your clothing, skin, or mucous membranes with potentially infectious materials. Here is one example. **Remove all PPE before exiting the patient room** except a respirator, if worn. Remove the respirator **after** leaving the patient room and closing the door. Remove PPE in the following sequence.

1. GLOVES

- Outside of gloves are contaminated!
- If your hands get contaminated during glove removal, immediately wash your hands or use an alcohol based hand sanitizer
- Using a gloved hand, grasp the palm area of the other gloved hand and peel off first glove
- Hold removed glove in gloved hand
- Slide fingers of ungloved hand under remaining glove at wrist and peel off second glove over first glove
- Discard gloves in a waste container

2. GOGGLES OR FACE SHIELD

- Outside of goggles or face shield are contaminated!
- If your hands get contaminated during goggle or face shield removal, immediately wash your hands or use an alcohol based hand sanitizer
- Remove goggles or face shield from the back by lifting head band or ear pieces
- If the item is reusable, place in designated receptacle for reprocessing. Otherwise, discard in a waste container

3. GOWN

- Gown front and sleeves are contaminated!
- If your hands get contaminated during gown removal, immediately wash your hands or use an alcohol based hand sanitizer
- Unfasten gown ties, taking care that sleeves don't contact your body when reaching for ties
- Pull gown away from neck and shoulders, touching inside of gown only
- Turn gown inside out
- Fold or roll into a bundle and discard in a waste container

4. MASK OR RESPIRATOR

- Front of mask/respirator is contaminated — DO NOT TOUCH!
- If your hands get contaminated during mask/respirator removal, immediately wash your hands or use an alcohol based hand sanitizer
- Grasp bottom ties or elastics of the mask/respirator, then the ones at the top, and remove without touching the front
- Discard in a waste container

5. WASH HANDS OR USE AN ALCOHOL-BASED HAND SANITIZER IMMEDIATELY AFTER REMOVING ALL PPE

OR

PERFORM HAND HYGIENE BETWEEN STEPS IF HANDS BECOME CONTAMINATED AND IMMEDIATELY AFTER REMOVING ALL PPE

CDC

Figure 5 Sequence for Doffing

Administrative and Environmental Protocols for Healthcare Facilities

Moreover, to protect the healthcare team further, healthcare facilities must provide strict guidelines pertaining to onsite management on the safe use of PPE along with implementing administrative and environmental controls. Continuous

19

checks and monitoring via observation and the presence of trained personnel during PPE Donning and doffing processes is, therefore, a must. Some of these processes are as follows.

1. Coordination and collaboration between the facility's prevention management system and occupational health department.
   √ Establishment and implementation of triage protocols to identify Ebola patients.
   √ Designate managers on site to oversee and monitor the implementation of standard precautions and protocols. This also includes administrating whether the provision of the Ebola treatment is safe and effective, i.e. observation of protocols before and after any staff member enters and exists an isolation and treatment area.
2. Training of nurses and healthcare team on all recommended protocols, including donning and doffing. These should be demonstrated during the training processes competency via testing. Trained observers on spot can also guide nurses and all members of the healthcare team to follow a step-by-step guide during donning and doffing PPE.
3. Designation of specific areas for donning and doffing in the facility. In addition, adequate provision of time must be allocated for this procedure without any disturbances and interruptions.
4. Ensuring practical precautions being implemented such as keeping hands away from the face and mouth area, limiting touching of surfaces and body fluids, avoiding contact of the skin with an Ebola patient, frequent disinfection of gloves, and wiping down of contaminated surfaces with alcohol-based disinfectant wipes.
5. Regular cleaning of patient care areas by nurses and physicians as part

of patient care guidelines to limit cross contamination to other parts of the facility.

6. Streamline a management plan that addresses decontamination and follow up of what to do if a healthcare worker comes in contact with an Ebola patient without protective equipment.

7. Observation of nurses, healthcare workers and doctors in the patient care area via video links or installation of glass walls.

ENSURING SAFETY OF PATIENTS

While the safety and protection of nurses and the healthcare team are taken into strict consideration, the safety of patients too needs to be ensured at the most. The earlier the diagnosis along with the execution of basic healthcare intervention, the better the chances of recovery and survival are.

Patients that are suspected of having the Ebola Virus or are diagnosed/undergoing treatment require isolation from other patients. Specific protocols and guidelines need to be followed in this regard. Some of them can be broken down as follows.

Patient Placement:
It is a standard practice that the patient having been diagnosed with the Ebola virus should be placed in a single patient room in isolation. The doors of the patient's room are to be closed at all times. In addition, the room is to be equipped with a private bathroom.

To make sure entry of nurses, healthcare professionals, and doctors is kept minimal, security personnel can be placed at the patient's door. They can ensure the PPE is worn by nurses and health care professionals in an appropriate and consistent manner while entering and exiting. Also, entry into the patient's room should be only during times of need. Visitor movement inside the facility should also be restricted and limited. A ledger that documents visit entries during essential needs should be maintained as well.

In addition, healthcare facilities should also maintain and keep a record of all health care professionals entering into the patient's room. This can help in tracing and tracking people that have come in contact with the patient along with the contact time in case any one of them contracts the virus.

Patient Care Equipment:

To ensure the safety of the patient, nurses, healthcare workers, and doctors, the use of dedicated medical equipment is essential. If possible, disposable medical equipment should be used to mitigate the risk of transferring the virus.

Similarly, if the medical equipment is not disposable or in a limited amount, then following the proper guidelines and protocols for cleaning and disinfection by central supply staff should be followed. It is better to follow the guidelines as per the manufactures instructions or the hospital policy in this regard to ensure proper sanitation and sterilization of the equipment.

Patient Care Considerations:

To mitigate the pain inflicted on the patient, it is best to limit the use of needles, other sharp objects, and equipment on the patient as much as possible. Taking of blood samples for laboratory testing, phlebotomy and medical procedures should be conducted only when necessary and for essential diagnostic evaluation. Limiting this to the minimum necessary for medical care along with safe injection practice is recommended by experts as well.

Apart from this, all needles and medical equipment used on the patient should be handled with care and disposed of in sealed and puncture-proof containers. This is an essential protocol that should be followed to minimize the spread of the Ebola Virus.

Basic Health Interventions:

The earlier the diagnosis and treatment, the better the survival and recovery rate is. Thus it is important to follow the basic health interventions in place. This includes ensuring the patient is well hydrated at all times, has access to oxygen in case oxygen levels or blood pressure drops, along with immediate treating of infection and ailments as they occur.

Regular cleaning, sterilization, and disinfection of patient care areas and sur-faces are also essential. This is to be carried out by the nurses and healthcare professionals entering the patient's rooms. Even absent visible contamination requires effective sanitization and cleaning.

Aerosol Generation Procedures (AGP)

It is recommended to avoid Aerosol Generation Procedures (AGP) for patients with Ebola Virus. If needed, it can be conducted with a combination of measures to re-duce occupational exposure. This includes the absence of all visitors during the procedure. Similarly, only those nurses and health care professionals needed are to be present that are essential and required for patient care and support.

The procedure should be conducted in a private room with doors kept closed. Before and after the procedure, entry and exit of the patient rooms should be minimum.

Ideally, an Airborne Infection Isolation Room (AIIR) is better suited for this purpose. Once conducted, proper doffing and sanitization procedures should be followed by all health care professionals that were present during the procedure. In addition, environmental surface cleaning and sanitization should also be followed.

MONITORING AND MANAGEMENT
OF POTENTIALLY EXPOSED PERSONNEL

Even with the strict adherence to the safety and protection guidelines, the chances of nurses, healthcare workers, and personnel contracting the virus are not eliminated entirely. In case of potential exposure, several steps can be taken to mitigate the risks. A systematic and well- organized approach towards the implementation of this procedure is essential.

It can be broken down as follows:

- √ Development of monitoring and management systems/policies by healthcare facilities.

- √ Sick leave policies for health care professionals should be flexible and in line with public health care guidance. All health care professionals should be made aware of these policies.

- √ Nurses, healthcare professionals, and others health care providers who come in contact with Ebola patients' blood, bodily fluids, or excretions should stop working immediately.

- √ Health supervisors should be contacted for an assessment and post exposure management services. This includes getting testing for all appropriate pathogens such as Hepatitis C, Human Immunodeficiency Virus (HIV), etc.

- √ Seeking immediate medical evaluation and testing along with strict isolation should follow.

√ It is important for the healthcare facility to notify the state health department in such cases.

√ Asymptomatic healthcare professionals should also isolate and receive medical evaluations twice a day for at least three weeks.

Apart from this, it is important for hospital and healthcare facilities to monitor potential symptoms and document any new developments that exposed personnel may be having.

EBOLA VIRUS - PROTOCOLS FOR DISINFECTION

The presence of Ebola virus strains in medical waste, on surfaces, and items is a cause of alarm, especially since the transmission rate for this disease is un-matched. Effective and efficient waste management of Ebola waste is a key element that aids towards its containment. And, it is also a vital requirement for ensuring a protective environment. In this regard, the physical and chemical agents needed to eradicate the virus can be highlighted as follows.

Physical Agents Used to Eradicate the Survivability of the Ebola Virus

Ebola virus, like other forms of bacteria, virus, and pathogens, can be eradicated via the use of heat, ultraviolet light, Gamma rays and even sunlight. Various methods ranging from heating materials that may have come in contact with the virus form medical waste to a temperature of 60°C (140°F) for an hour to heating 80°C (176°F) for half an hour can be sufficient. In addition, submerging the infected item in hot water for five minutes can also be done to kill the virus.

Similarly, an autoclave can also be used for this purpose, given it is followed as per its due waste cycle. Incineration is another method used to kill the Ebola virus present on large items such as hospital beds or mattresses. The ash and debris left over in the end once incineration is completed does not contain the microbial pathogens, thus making it safe for disposal.

Chemical Agents Used to Eradicate the Survivability of the Ebola Virus

Apart from using physical methods of Ebola virus waste disposal, chemical elements are also used. Some of the most common chemical agents are bleach, alcohol, halogens, peroxide, ammonia, detergents, and phenolic. They are effective and can be easily found in high-grade disinfectants designed for medical institutions. They are also used to sanitize areas frequently touched in the patient's room to prevent further transmission. In addition, disinfectants are also recommended to be added to bagged and sealed waste.

EBOLA VIRUS -
PROTOCOLS FOR SAFE DISPOSAL OF MEDICAL WASTE

Waste management of Ebola associated waste is a top priority for hospitals and medical facilities. Here are some of the practices carried out to ensure safe handling of the waste generated via patient care. They can be demarcated into three areas.

The first aspect rests on the containments and safe packaging of the waste. Keeping waste close to where the waste has been generated from is the safest option in this regard. This aspect of primary packaging waste is crucial going forward. Re-opening containers once the waste has been sealed is another added feature that ensures effective containment of the virus.

Second on the list is limited access into the patient's room while waste is amidst the process of packaging. And the last is the proper use of personal protective equipment while handling Ebola associated waste. Whether this waste is to be inactivated within the hospital or medical facility or transported to a secondary location for offsite inactivation, is to be determined by the medical facility itself.

In most cases, a waste management team is organized for the job of inactivation. With proper guidelines regarding bagging, packaging, transporting, and disinfecting the waste, a systematic and strategic approach gets the job done effectively. If onsite inactivation is the protocol being followed, then incineration or autoclave may be the approach deployed. For inactivation away from point of waste generation, compliance with guidelines for packaging and transport are to be followed strictly.

In addition, certain guidelines can be kept in mind to ensure the safety of nurses, the healthcare team and providers. They can be defined as follows.

√ Avoid overfilling of waste bags. It is recommended to seal and close bags once they are two-thirds full.

√ For storage of Ebola associated waste within the patient's room till transportation for inactivation, primary closure procedures for solid waste bags and objects are to be followed as prescribed.

√ For storage outside of the patient's room, primary and secondary closure procedures are to be followed.

Primary Closure Procedures

To ensure primary closure procedures of Ebola associated waste, solid waste can be identified. This can range from any item falling under the category of medical equipment, linens, dressings, injections, portable toilets, emesis pans, used personal protective equipment by the medical staff, or by products from the cleaning processes. No matter what, all staff from nurses to EVS must observe these precautions.

These items require double bagging that is carried out inside the patient's room. The supplies required for the packaging of Ebola associated waste include leak-proof bags that are biohazardous. These bags are to be lined inside waste containers. Bags are also to be sealed in a way that reduces the risk of it being punctured or torn. Tying a goose-neck knot at the neck of the bag is an appropriate method that is followed.

For waste devoid of sharp objects and requiring autoclaving for inactivation of the virus, a sufficient amount of water or liquid is added to the primary bag. For inactivation that is to be conducted offsite, adding liquid may not be required.

And, lastly, disinfection of the outside surface of the secondary bag along with storage of the sealed bags in a designated area for transport is to follow suit.

Secondary Closure Procedures

Once the waste has undergone its primary closure procedure, wiping down of the exterior surface of the double-bagged waste is carried out by healthcare providers. The outer lid of the container in which the bagged waste is to be placed is to be secured tight. This is then to be placed in its designated area for onsite or offsite inactivation.

From here on, reopening of the container or transport cart in which the bagged waste is loaded is strictly not allowed. The personnel that is part of the waste management team are also required to wear personal protective equipment at all times as per protocol. Transportation to a waste vendor approved pickup, and further secure storage is then ensured.

In this manner, the effective storage, transportation, and disposal of Ebola associated waste are ensured by nurses, health care professionals, and doctors.

EBOLA VIRUS -
PROTOCOLS FOR HANDLING LIQUID WASTE

Liquid waste produced in medical facilities requires an even more meticulous approach for disposal. This is because the patient's waste is a petri dish for the Ebola virus. And coming in contact with any liquid waste can lead to droplet transmission of the virus at a rate higher than from touching contaminated surfaces.

To effectively dispose of liquid waste, pretreatment may be required. This is especially the case if sanitary sealed containers may be at risk of being damaged or broken. Therefore, strict adherence to the protocols for handling liquid waste is an essential requirement. They can be broken down as follows.

1. Primary handling of this liquid waste is required by nurses, healthcare providers, and doctors present in the room. It is also important to wear personal protective equipment while handling any liquid waste.

2. To start off, liquid waste is to be disposed off in the toilet from a low level—this is to avoid the liquid waste from splashing and contaminating the area around.

3. After this is done, the lid is to be closed before flushing. This prevents any contaminated waste from spreading.

4. Cleaning and disinfecting of the flush handle, seat, lid, and nearby surfaces using hospital-grade disinfectant are to be carried out.

5. Cleaning cloths are to be discarded in leak-proof biohazard bags following primary closure procedures.

6. Emesis and portable toilet equipment are to be discarded as per solid waste disposal protocols.

7. Once the liquid waste has been discarded and the affected areas have been sanitized, proper sanitation of the personal protective equipment follow by doffing is to be followed.

In case of spillage:

While following this procedure requires careful handling and attention, there may be times where spillage may occur. If this happens, the protocol for handling spills can be followed. Here is how the spillage of blood or any other infectious waste can be cleaned up and is disposed of effectively.

1. Spillage management is to be carried out by nurses, health care providers, and doctors present while having the personal protective equipment worn at all times.

2. It is then important to isolate the area where the spillage has occurred. Any other healthcare provides or individuals are not allowed to ensure the patents room or impacted area till disinfection has been completed.

3. A solidifier or absorbent material is to be placed on top of the spillage. After this, the relevant disinfectant is to be poured over. This is to rest there for a sufficient period of time as per the manufacturer's instructions for spillage management.

4. Use of absorbent disposable towels can then be used to help remove the spill. This is to be immediately disposed of in a leak-proof biohazard bag, following primary closure procedures as recommended.

5. A hospital disinfectant is to be applied after this step, allowing it to rest. Once done, the area can be wiped using disposable cleaning materials.

6. The disposal of the materials used for cleaning the spill is to be handled according to the solid waste disposal guidelines.

7. Lastly, sanitization of the soiled personal protective equipment along with the doffing procedure is to be followed.

Preventing spillage from occurring while conducting patient care is a step that is always recommended. This includes various steps such as providing the patient with a large biohazard bag if they are feeling nauseous. This will help in containing any emesis and keeping the surrounding areas protected from possible contamination. Similarly, if the patient is experiencing dysentery, then they can be wrapped in an impermeable sheet to prevent cross contamination.

PROTOCOLS FOR EMERGENCY MEDICAL SERVICES (EMS) – PREHOSPITALIZATION PROTOCOLS

With an outbreak in Ebola virus cases, local and state authorities are to be alerted by hospital management. Alongside, there may be instances where potential Ebola virus patients may require assessment and transportation to the hospital. In this case, there is a specific set of guidelines that is to be followed.

Patient Screening and Assessment

To reduce contact transmission of the virus, the Emergency Medical Services (EMS) provider should only approach the Patient Under Investigation (PUI) while being covered in personal protective equipment. This is to be worn before entering the area where the PUI is present and is to be removed when no longer in contact with the PUI. Proper donning and doffing protocols are to be followed under the supervision of a trained officer for this procedure.

In addition, it is advisable for the EMS provider to maintain a social distancing of at least three feet from the PUI while conducting the initial screening. This along with an assessment of the patient's travel history is to be taken. This includes the area of recent travel or having come in contact with the blood or body fluids of another PUI or patient confirmed with the Ebola virus. The PUI is to be questioned about the symptoms or signs of the Ebola virus such as fever, weakness, abdominal pain, emesis, etc.

It is also important to note that if the EMS providers unprotected skin comes in contact with the PUI's blood or bodily fluid, then they are required to wash the affected area using an antiseptic solution and stop working. Informing the relevant authorities about the exposure to a PUI is to be conveyed followed by immediate care and isolation to monitor any symptom development.

Patient Management

For EMs providers, managing the patient before hospitalization can be challenging. The risk of exposure to the Ebola virus here is high, especially since the illness can cause staggering, delirium, and erratic behavior in the PUI. During this process, minimizing contact with others is essential. The PUI is to be kept separate in another room until the diagnosis is completed.

Limiting the use of needles and sharp objects along with proper disposal of liquid and solid waste is to be conducted by the EMS provider wearing the personal protective equipment at all times. In addition, oral medication for nausea can be administered as per the medical directors' guidance and prescription.

Large procedures such as resuscitation procedures are advisable not to be executed in the absence of a safe and controlled environment, i.e. the patient's home or moving vehicle. They can be conducted when arriving at the hospital. This is because these procedures including open suctioning of airways, endotracheal intubation, and cardiopulmonary resuscitation result in a large amount of bodily fluid being lost.

Prehospital Care of PUI

The principles of personal protective equipment are to be followed by the EMS providers in strict adherence. This is because prehospital care is often conducted in an uncontrolled environment such as the home, thus bringing up additional operational procedures and challenges.

While transporting the patient, the EMS providers that have come in contact with the PUI are required to remain at the back of the ambulance and avoid driving. A designated driver may be chosen for this purpose, ensuring that the patient compartment is in isolation from where they are driving.

While the PUI is being transported, all nonessential items and materials are to be kept separate and away from the PUI. This is to minimize the risk of contamination. The stretcher too is required to be covered with an impermeable material before the patient is placed. Ensuring these guidelines are followed along with proper donning and doffing procedures is essential in containing the spread of the Ebola virus.

Transportation of the Patient Under Investigation to a Healthcare Facility

If the PUI is experiencing aggressive symptoms and has a confirmed history of exposure to the Ebola virus, then it is suggested that they be transported to the nearest medical facility immediately. This is to further evaluate and analyze the symptoms and condition of the patient. The transportation procedure is to be followed as per the pre defined protocols at hand. These are developed by the hospital, healthcare team, EMS providers, and public health officials. Thus, their strict adherence is a requirement for all representatives involved in the PUI's transportation.

To begin with, isolating the ambulance driver from the compartment where the patient is placed is important. In addition, hospital-grade disinfectants are to be present in the form of spray bottles or wipes. These two aspects are the first on the checklist before loading the patient into the ambulance. If the patient requires medical assistance on route to the medical facility, then EMS providers present are advised to do so while keeping the following guidelines in mind.

Infection Control

To limit contact with the PUI and ensure safety for all EMS providers, appropriate use of personal protective equipment is required. The presence of a trained observer for ensuring proper donning and doffing procedures is essential here. This is to be followed by a limit in activities, especially procedures that are invasive during transportation. This is because conducting medical procedures on the route can increase the risk of exposure to the Ebola virus.

Similarly, the use of needles and sharp objects are to be limited as well. These items are required careful handling by the EMS providers and require proper disposal in sealed and puncture-proof biohazard bags.

Documentation

Written documentation of patient care provided is to be provided by the EMS providers after the patient has reached the medical facility and the ambulance has been disinfected. This written documentation is to match the verbal account of patient care provided by the EMS providers while handing over the patient to the emergency department.

The documentation should also consist of the response and contact level of the EMS providers with the PUI for further evaluation purposes. This record is to be used by the medical staff, nurses, doctors, and healthcare team in the medical facility and need not be shared with other local public healthcare authorities.

Disinfecting the Transport Vehicle after PUI Handover

Once the PUI has been transported to the relevant medical facility, disinfecting the ambulance is important. This is to ensure the safety of the EMS providers and the next patient that would be traveling in the ambulance. The guidelines and steps that are required to be conducted are as follows.

1. Cleaning and disinfection of the ambulance are to be carried out by the EMS providers in areas where the PUI has come in contact. This also includes areas where the PUI's bodily fluids are present, i.e. emesis, sweat, blood, diarrhea, or blood. To clean up, the wearing of personal protective equipment is a must. However, if there are no signs of bodily fluids present, then a face shield, surgical mask, impermeable gown, and gloves can be worn instead.

2. A hospital-grade and certified disinfectant are to be used to wipe down are areas of concern. These include patient care surfaces such as the stretcher, door handles, flooring, walls, work surfaces, and medical equipment present in the vehicle. Other areas suspected of being infected are required thorough disinfection to minimize the risk of virus transmission.

3. For spillage and the presence of bodily fluids from the PUI, careful measures are to be followed. For this, wearing personal protective equipment is essential. Removal of the spillage matter, cleaning of the soiled site, and disinfection are to be followed as per the protocol of handling liquid waste mentioned previously. A potent chemical agent is to be used to overcome the presence of protein in bodily fluids. The disinfection procedure as per the manufacture's guidelines is to be executed hereafter and all infected materials and items used for disinfection are to be disposed off in puncture proof and sealed biohazard bags as per primary closure procedures.

4. If any of the reusable equipment aboard the ambulance is contaminated such as the C, then they are required to be placed in biohazard bags for further disinfection. All other items are required to be cleaned

according to the manufacturer's guidelines while ensuring personal protective equipment is worn at all times.

5. To ensure even more care and mitigation of cross contamination, any infected cloth products, linens, and non-fluid impermeable pillows can be discarded at the medical facility. This may even be followed for mattresses that may have been utilized without having a plastic or impermeable covering.

Follow Up Procedures by EMS Providers after Tending to Ebola Virus Patient

Reporting measures along with a follow-up of the PUI is important for the EVD providers. This is in case the PUI is diagnosed with the Ebola virus that is highly contagious and potent. It is recommended that policies for monitoring EMS providers are set in place, especially for those that may have potentially been exposed to the Ebola virus during the patient assessment, care, or transportation.

For this, special policies including sick leaves for EMS providers can be developed and implemented. It is preferred that the policies be flexible, and in alignment with public health orders and guidelines. In addition, all EMS providers including the nurses and health care team at the medical facilities that provide daily services are to be made aware of these sick leave policies.

Any healthcare provider, including nurses and doctors, that have come in contact with the bodily fluids, excretions, or secretions of an Ebola Virus patient should stop working effectively immediately. This is to be followed by practicing hand hygiene, washing all skin surfaces with an antiseptic solution, and irrigating all mucous membranes such as the eyes and mouth with water. Healthcare supervisors are to then be contacted and informed for immediate assessment and monitoring followed by isolation. Follow-up care and medical evaluation are then to be carried out as per hospital policies.

Transportation of Pediatric Patients Under Investigation

Concerns often arise about the protocols needed for the safe transportation of children and adolescents under the age of 18. These are for patients that may have been diagnosed with the Ebola virus or still be under investigation.

For such pediatric patients, transportation via pediatric transport is recommended. However, if the facility and services required for children are not present, then the following aspects can be ensured in place. The EMS's child restraint system may also be applied along with the presence of basic and advanced life support needs for children.

Isopods or pediatric isolation transport units are an option that can be opted for by EMS providers while transportation. This is essentially a piece of equipment designed to allow air circulation or negative pressure and access that can accommodate up to three individuals. The purchase of isopods is at the discretion of the medical facility and they often come equipped with IV pumps and stretchers. In addition, the use of the child care seat can be used too. It is preferred that this car seat be the child's car seat and is deposited at the receiving facility for disinfection and decontamination.

Can the Child Be Accompanied?

The child must be transported alone. This is despite the standard protocol of a child being assisted by a caregiver due to the high risk of transmission and contamination. However, a caregiver may accompany given that the child is not experiencing any form of emesis, secretion, or excretion and if symptoms are mild.

Ensuring Use of Personal Protective Equipment

It is required that the caregiver be a parent or legal guardian. If neither is present, the permission of a designated adult may be taken from the former to assist the child. Just like the EMS providers are required to wear personal protective equipment, the caregiver or adult accompanying the minor is also required to use appropriate personal protective equipment. A face shield, impermeable surgical gown, face mask, and gloves are essential requirements here. A trained observer is to be present here to ensure the proper protocols for donning and doffing by the caregiver are carried out. Children, on the other hand, are not required to wear personal protective equipment. This is because the personal protective equipment is aimed at protecting the person wearing it from being exposed to the pathogen. It is not intended to contain the patient's bodily fluids. Also, covering the child may interfere with the patient assessment process being conducted.

Decontamination and Patient Care

Moreover, invasive procedures along with the use of needles and sharp objects during transportation are to be performed at the minimum. This will ensure the child is not agitated and restless during transportation. Once the vehicle or ambulance has arrived at the facility, the decontamination plan is to be executed as per standard practice.

PROTOCOLS FOR SCREENING AND CARE
OF PREGNANT WOMEN WITH EBOLA VIRUS DISEASE

Ebola virus can manifest itself in more dangerous ways in women that are pregnant. Limited evidence does suggest that women who are expecting are more at risk from facing severe symptoms and mortality rates. There may also be fetal loss and hemorrhage in some cases. There have been many infants born to women with the Ebola virus that have not survived. The cause of death has however not been ruled out because autopsy is not done on Ebola patients.

There has however been one reported case of an infant born to a woman with the Ebola virus who has survived. The mother contracted the virus eight days before her delivery and was provided with basic intervention facilities. This included favipiravir that was administered on her fifth day of diagnosis. She, unfortunately, died on the eighth day after spontaneous delivery. The infant was treated with a buffy coat transfusion from a previous Ebola virus survivor, along with monoclonal antibodies and anti-viral medications. The infant experienced no symptoms of the Ebola virus except seizures and had a normal developmental and growth cycle when monitored twelve months later.

Nevertheless, the possibility of the Ebola virus being transmitted into the fetus is present. This is because the Ebola virus can permeate through the placenta. The RNA of the Ebola virus has been detected in the amniotic fluid, umbilical cord, and vaginal secretions of pregnant women. They have also been present in the fetal meconium and buccal swab of neonates. The Ebola virus strains have also persisted in the amniotic fluid post-recovery. Thus, placing infection control and care of the mother as a priority.

On the other hand, women who have contracted the Ebola virus and recovered have not had any issues conceiving. Nor has there been any risk of transmission to the fetus when getting pregnant post-recovery.

Screening and Treatment for Pregnant Women with the Ebola Virus

To ensure proper screen and assessment of pregnant women, it is important to document the mothers' travel history and exposure to a potential Ebola virus patient within the last 21 days. Assessing for signs and symptoms such as fever, and diarrhea is to be followed next.

If symptoms of the Ebola virus are visible, immediate isolation is to be conducted of the patient followed by medical management and basic intervention. If there are no symptoms but the pregnant woman has certainly been exposed to an Ebola virus patient, then assessment of other epidemiologic risks is to be conducted. This also includes obstetric care that focuses on early treatment of any hemorrhage. It is important to note that spontaneous abortions, high perinatal mortality rates, and intrapartum hemorrhage are common among women with the Ebola virus disease.

Labor and Delivery Procedures for Pregnant Women Having the Ebola Virus

For women that are pregnant and have a confirmed case of the Ebola virus, infection control during labor and delivery is important. This is because the delivery room and labor units in the medical facility or hospital are subject to exposure to blood and bodily fluids from the amniotic sac of the mother. This places the nurses, healthcare team, and doctors at high risk of being exposed to the Ebola virus.

Thus, personal protective equipment is an essential requirement that is to be worn by all individuals present in the delivery room. This is to be as per the recommended donning procedure followed by all healthcare workers while caring for PUI's and patients diagnosed with the Ebola virus.

In addition, pregnant nurses and healthcare workers are advised to maintain distance from pregnant women diagnosed with the Ebola virus. They should only provide basic health intervention measures or care. This is because of the risks of contracting the virus that can impact maternal and fetal health. Similarly, the restrictive personal protective equipment may be uncomfortable and distressing for pregnant nurses and healthcare workers as well.

Method of Delivery to Keep in Consideration

There is no preferred method of delivery for a pregnant woman that has been diagnosed with the Ebola virus. In addition, the method of delivery has no direct impact on fetal loss as well. Causes of neonatal loss have not been ruled out and research on this phenomenon is still underway. However, the possibility of perinatal death due to transplacental viral passage or transmission is a factor that can be taken into consideration.

All in all, the method that is used for delivering the fetus is at the discretion of the medical facility. Regardless of it being a cesarean or vaginal delivery, it is to be equipped with the appropriate protocols and procedures for minimizing blood loss along with strict adherence to wearing personal protective equipment. Contingency plans for what steps are to be followed in case of severe postpartum hemorrhage are to be set beforehand as well. This is also to be followed by the guidelines set in place for disinfecting and cleaning the delivery room or labor unit.

Handling Visitors for Laboring Patients

Visitors are to be strictly not allowed to visit the patient or baby with the Ebola virus. Some exceptions may be considered such as in the case of the patient's spouse or father of the child. If a support person is required during labor, then this may be allowed after assessing the risks and benefits. This coupled with any other visits to the hospital are to be recorded, monitored, and controlled. Scheduling of visits along with their management lies in the hospital procedures and protocols. If possible, video conferencing with the patient can be arranged to avoid in-person visitation and ensure safety for everyone.

However, if in-person visitation does take place, then the risk category needs to be identified. The visitors too need to be screened before entering the patient's room. A healthcare professional should also be present to ensure there is no contact with the patient. The visitor is to be properly covered in personal protective equipment as per the donning procedures. Once the visit is over, the visitor is to be trained to safely remove the personal protective equipment and be monitored after. These measures are important in order to prevent the risk of infection and transmission from occurring.

Breastfeeding Recommendations for Mothers with the Ebola Virus

Concerns often arise about whether the Ebola virus can be transferred into the baby via the mother's breast milk if she has been diagnosed with the Ebola virus. Studies have confirmed the presence of the Ebola virus in breast milk, however, the duration of its presence along with the estimated time of it being cleared from the breast milk has yet not been confirmed. As per researchers, the presence of the Ebola virus strain may linger on in breast milk for 6 to 26 days on the onset of the disease.

Thus, it is recommended that women who are positive for the Ebola virus or have recently recovered should avoid breastfeeding. Testing of breast milk can be conducted where available though. The genetic material of the Ebola virus can be detected via various tests, thus making it useful in deciding whether the mother can return to breastfeeding her child or not.

If a mother is under investigation for the Ebola virus, it is advisable for her to not breastfeed. Donor milk can be provided as a substitute for the infant instead. To maintain the process of lactation, the mother may use a dedicated breast pump to pump out the breast milk. This should be done in isolation and within the designated patient's room. Similarly, careful handling of this breast milk is to be carried out. This bodily fluid is considered infectious and is to be disposed off as per waste management guidelines. In addition, the breast pump is to not be used by any other patient.

On the other hand, there is no known risk of the Ebola virus being transmitted to the infant born to a woman who becomes pregnant after recovering from the Ebola virus. Thus, breastfeeding is recommended and is safe for healthy infantile development in such cases.

Taking Care of Neonates Born to Women with the Ebola Virus

Since it isn't confirmed if all neonates born to mothers with Ebola contract the virus, the neonates delivered of mothers with confirmed cases are to be considered as PUI's. In cases where the neonate survives, they are to be immediately separated from the mother. They are then to be given care in isolation for 21 days and monitored for any symptom development. Non-invasive screening tests can be administered by healthcare professionals while wearing personal protective equipment.

Invasive procedures along with immunizations and circumcision too should be delayed until 21 days of isolation and active monitoring have been completed. Blood specimen tests can then be conducted to rule out whether the neonate has a negative result for the Ebola virus. In addition, if the infant shows any symptoms of illness or becomes febrile while being hospitalized, other causes of such occurrences should be considered. These include possible viral illnesses and bacterial infections that could be acquired from the hospital environment.

HANDLING SPECIMENS AND
INFECTION CONTROL FOR EBOLA VIRUS DISEASE

To ensure the safe handling of specimens, following the standards and protocols established is important. This starts with the use of wearing personal protective equipment while handling all types of blood or potentially infectious elements. The standards that are compliant with the OSHA blood borne pathogens standard and can be broken down into different aspects.

Risk assessment for the specimens is a task that the laboratory director or biosafety officer is required to determine. The potential bioaerosols, splashes, or sprays generated from the procedures conducted in the laboratory are included during this process. The Ebola virus may enter or come into contact with the laboratorian's mucous membranes, eyes, and skin. Thus, the required personal protective equipment is to then be adjusted and safety protocols are to be updated to ensure the personnel or healthcare team present in the laboratory is protected.

Similarly, the healthcare provider who is collecting the specimens from a patient that is diagnosed with the Ebola virus or is under investigation is required to wear appropriate personal protective equipment. This extends to hospital-grade gloves, a face shield, mask, and goggles to cover the eyes and mouth, along with a water-resistant gown.

Laboratory Testing Guidelines
The person testing the specimen is required to ensure personal protective equipment is worn at all times. This too includes the hospital-grade gloves, a face shield, mask, and goggles to cover the eyes and mouth, along with a water-resistant gown.

For additional precaution, a Class II Biosafety cabinet or Plexiglas splash guard is required. This further ensures safety and protection for the person conducting the testing of the specimens. Moreover, the safety measures for laboratory instruments are to be used as per manufacturer guidelines.

The disinfection and cleaning of surfaces where specimens are being tested and processed are applicable for laboratories. If a spill of the specimen occurs, using a potent disinfectant and following guidelines as in the case of spillage cleanup are to be followed immediately. Hospital- grade disinfectants are usually strong enough to kill the Ebola virus pathogen on surfaces as the Ebola virus is an enveloped virus. This means they are not resistant to disinfectants and can easily be deactivated using hospital-grade disinfectants.

Laboratory Waste Management

The Department of Transportation (DOT) has classified the Ebola virus as a Category A infection. This means that the substance is required to be packaged and transported as per the DOT's Hazardous Materials Regulations (HMR). Here all materials and items used such as sharp objects, linens, soiled dressings, emesis pans, portable toilets, respirators, and personal protective equipment are to be considered as a Category A substance. This means that the material and substances are infectious.

Thus, the waste generated while testing the specimen in the laboratory is required to be placed in a leak-proof bio-hazard bag. To avoid contamination of the exterior surface of this bag, it is important to place this bag in a sealed waste container. It is advisable to provide autoclave or steam sterilization to deactivate the virus and reduce the volume of potentially infectious waste. For equipment and material that is disposed of in the sewer system, the guidelines put in place by the respective hospital and medical facility are to be followed.

This is because not all medical facilities may be equipped with features needed to handle the disposal process and safely inactivate the infectious materials.

Collection and Transportation

The presence of the Ebola virus can be identified in the blood after symptoms have developed. The main one being fever. However, it may take up to three days after the symptom has developed that the Ebola virus can be effectively detected. Real-time RT-PCR tests three to ten days after the onset of the symptoms can thus be conducted to rule out the diagnosis.

For this, a minimum of 4 ml of the blood is to be drawn from the PUI. It is to be placed in a plastic collection tube. Glass or heparinized tubes are not recommended for Ebola virus specimen testing. In addition, the whole blood preserved with EDTA is preferred. The serum or plasma separation in the primary collection container is not necessary.

Once conducted, it is recommended that the specimen be placed in a durable and leak-proof bag for transportation to the laboratory. A pneumatic tube system for the transportation of the specimen in the same facility is not advisable as it may increase the risk of leak or breakage. The specimen is to then be stored at 2-8°C. if this facility is not available, cold packs can be used to keep the specimen preserved at the ideal temperatures.

Diagnostic Testing of Specimen

To detect the Ebola virus in the blood specimen, various methods can be used. A real-time RT- PCR test is the ideal process followed that is to be conducted in a certified laboratory. Serologic testing is another option that can be followed to evaluate the presence of antibodies.

Packaging and Shipment of Specimens to Local Health Care Departments

While shipping and transporting specimens collected for Ebola virus testing, it is imperative that collection tubes are kept sealed. They are not to be opened till the relevant destination has been reached.

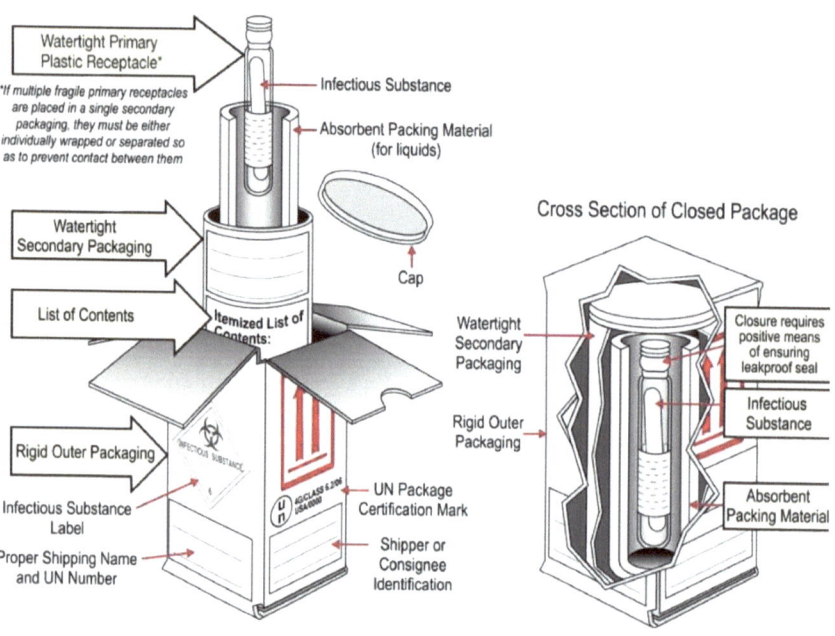

Figure 6 Packaging

Source: Centers for Disease Control and Prevention

The following steps are to be followed to ensure safe transportation and shipment.

1. Issuance of notification to relevant facility or health care department for the transportation of the specimen.

2. The tracking number is to be noted down before dispatching.

3. A triple packaging system is to be followed. This includes the primary packaging in a sealable bag combined with the wrapping of the specimen with absorbent material. Once done, a watertight and leak-proof container is to be used for final shipment.

4. Proper labeling of the specimen along with patient details is to be present.

5. Specification of specimen storage is to be provided on the outside of the container enclosing the specimen.

In case of any potential exposure to the specimen or any infectious material, immediate reporting to the relevant authorities is to be followed as per established protocols.

POLICIES AT HAND

A lot of efforts are being made to unearth the intricacies of the Ebola virus. Having faced this unwanted disease for decades has resulted in improved and better practices of containment and treatment. There have also been many efforts made to mitigate the adverse impacts of the Ebola virus by nurses, healthcare teams, and service providers alike. Some of the common protocols and guidelines that have received praise and are being followed earnestly can be identified.

Protocols for Traveling to an Area Affected by the Ebola Virus

If travel to such an area is essential, then practicing personal hygiene is important. Use of soap and water to wash hands frequently or the use of an alcohol-based sanitizer can help. The awareness of this combined with avoiding contact with any blood or bodily fluid of a person infected with the Ebola virus is also being efficiently disseminated to the general public by nurses, health care providers, and doctors.

- √ Avoid touching surfaces and items that could be potentially be infected. Door handles, clothes, money and medical equipment, etc. are some of them. If touched, washing or sanitizing of hands Is to be followed immediately.
- √ It is advisable to avoid attending funeral processions, religious rituals, and handling/touching the body of a person that has died from the Ebola virus.
- √ Stay updated and informed on areas impacted by the Ebola virus via the radio, television, or internet facility if available. Avoid visiting or traveling to these Ebola hotspots.
- √ Stay distant from nonhuman primates and bats. This includes their blood, raw meat, and excretions.

√   Follow controlled traveling guidelines

Once returned from an area affected by the Ebola virus, it is mandatory to observe isolation and quarantine for at least 21 days. During this period, it is important to avoid sharing personal items and practice self-monitoring (on their own or with delegated supervision/public health supervision) and self-observation of their health for any developing symptoms. An RT-PCR test on the blood specimen can then be conducted in conjunction with the local public health authorities as per standard protocol.

Isolation Unit Protocols for Medical Facilities
As stated previously, following the set guidelines and protocols for coming in contact with PUI's is to be followed earnestly. For infection control, designated isolation areas in medical facilities are crucial. However, these units are to be fully equipped with the desired resources, rules as regulations. Strict implementation of which is essential for Ebola virus containment. Here are the guidelines.

- Use of disposable materials and items is recommended. They should be non-porous and fluid impermeable to allow for effective cleaning and disinfection and are to be stored outside of the isolation area.
- Maintaining at least six feet between the PUI and health care professional is mandatory. Wearing personal protective equipment by nurses, healthcare teams, doctors and any relevant stakeholder entering the isolation unit is essential. Minimal contact with PUI's is to be observed. This is to help reduce exposure to potentially infected individuals.
- Essential supplies required for cleaning and disinfecting are to be kept inside the isolation areas.

- Limit the use of medical procedures that require needles and sharp objects as much as possible. If used, then this equipment is to be disposed off as per primary and secondary waste disposal procedures.
- Aerosol generating procedures along with those that can generate splashes of infectious material are to be avoided. For instance, transferring liquid waste or bodily fluid from one container to another is to be avoided and kept at minimal.
- Provision of materials and resources required for basic intervention is to be present in the isolation unit. Oxygen support along with mechanical ventilators are to be operational and provided to PUI as needed.
- Waste collection and disposal are to be followed as per protocols. Dry solid waste is to be collected in leak proof biohazard bags. The same goes for waste soaked with blood or bodily fluids. Handling of PUI's bodily fluids with utmost care is to be followed.
- Portable toilets, bedpans, or urinals are to be dedicated for each PUI whose lid is required to be kept closed when not in use. Emesis, feces, and urine are to be disposed off carefully while avoiding splashes and spills.

EBOLA EXPOSURE CONTROL PLAN – POLICY & PROCEDURE

To ensure the effective execution of the policies in place, an Ebola Exposure Control plan can be formulated taking into account the various elements surrounding employee and environmental health, safety, and infection prevention, etc. the aim of which is to identify analyze and observe the operations, tasks, and areas where nurses, healthcare service providers, doctors and employees at the medical facility are at a greater risk of being exposed to the Ebola virus.

It entails the work practices, protocols, and training provided to the professionals at stake to further streamline the plan at hand. In addition, it also provides nurses, healthcare teams, and doctors the opportunity to monitor the effectiveness of each procedure and policy and offer their valuable input toward updating and readjusting the policy as per changing circumstances.

This update is recommended to be made on an annual basis or whenever deemed necessary. This will help identify the gaps, address them going forward, and enable an environment of continuous improvement and performance along with a reflection of the innovation and changes accepted.

To ensure this process takes place in a streamlined and systematic manner, committees pertaining to each protocol are to be formulated. These committees are to then review and update the Ebola Exposure Control Plan and have it approved by the relevant authorities.

Exposure To Ebola Virus

Here is the comprehensive guide containing all health care personnel that are at high risk of exposure, the areas tasks, operations, procedures, and protocols that involve risk of exposure.

Employees at risk of exposure to the Ebola virus infection—via contact with PUIs, execution of basic health intervention procedures given to patients, or coming in contact with infectious materials.

1. Ebola Response Team – this includes the following:
   - Nurses
   - Physicians
   - Doctors
   - EMS personnel
   - Security Personnel that escort the PUI or patient
2. Nurses and physicians who enter the room where a PUI or patient confirmed with the Ebola virus is admitted
3. Surgical and Lab technicians that come in contact with a PUI or patient diagnosed with the Ebola virus
4. Patient Care Technicians who provide basic health intervention to Ebola patients
5. Radiology Technicians
6. Receptionists and personnel at the front desk of a medical facility
7. Employee Health Personnel who monitor employees that care for Ebola virus patients

Specific areas where there is a high risk of coming in contact with the Ebola virus are as follows:

- Outpatient Departments
- Urgent Care Units
- Emergency
- Isolation Units
- Labor And Delivery Units

The operations that involve risk of exposure are as follows:

Since the Ebola virus spread via bodily fluids, any procedure or activity that involves close proximity to the individual infected with the Ebola virus's broken skin, mucous membranes, secretions, etc. increases the risk of exposure. This includes escorting or transportation of the patient, providing patient care includes but is not limited to drawing blood, providing respiratory therapy, bathing and monitoring of overall health.

In addition, patient care extends to the following aspects:

- Cleaning, collecting, and disposing of infectious waste from a patient with the Ebola virus
- Disinfection of the medical equipment in the patient's room
- Handling of personal protective equipment after tending to a PUI or patient
- Handling and transportation of specimens collected from PUI or patients with the Ebola virus
- Entering the patient room to troubleshoot medical equipment, repair ventilation or other systems

Engineering Controls

To reduce employee exposure, engineering controls extend from having designated isolation rooms with ventilation systems in place to designated areas for donning and doffing personal protective equipment. Specified shower facilities for the nurses, healthcare team and doctors are also to be included here.

It is recommended for the isolation room to be equipped with the appropriate ventilation system. An Airborne Infection Isolation room is negatively pressured.

It comes with its bathroom attached or portable toilet as deemed fit. Thus, they are ideal for aerosol-generating procedures.

Work Practices

Protocols set in place to diagnose, isolate and care for patients with the Ebola virus are to be followed as per the policies set by the medical facility. Workflows are to be designed and executed systematically while having personal protective equipment worn as needed.

These practices include:

- Identification and diagnosis of the patient
- Isolation of Ebola patients or PUIs
- Alerting relevant authorities
- Provision of basic intervention to the patient
- Protection of nurses, healthcare teams, and doctors by ensuring proper procedure of donning and doffing personal protective equipment is followed
- Waste management protocols
- Specimen collection, transportation, and assessment protocols
- Aerosol generating procedures to be followed as per guidelines set in place
- Cleaning and disinfection of patient room
- Medical evaluation and monitoring of nurses, health care teams, and doctors

Medical Services

In case of employee exposure, Employee Health Services and relevant authorities are to assist with monitoring the employee's symptoms. The risk categories are to be defined and labeled as high-risk exposures, low-risk exposures to no identifiable risk.

High-risk exposures include:

- Contact with Ebola patient's mucous membranes, blood, or bodily fluids without having worn personal protective equipment
- Contact with the dead body of Ebola patient
- Residing in a home or facility where an Ebola patient is present
- Having come in contact with an Ebola patient during home care without proper personal protective equipment
- Breach in personal protective equipment while near an Ebola patient
- Close contact with an Ebola patient for a prolonged period of time without personal protective equipment

Low-risk exposures include:

- Being present in an area where there has been an Ebola outbreak
- Having come in contact with a symptomatic person with the Ebola virus for a brief period of time
- Traveled in a vehicle or aircraft with a person having Ebola who was symptomatic

No identified risk includes:

- Coming in contact with an asymptomatic person with the Ebola virus
- Contact with a person having Ebola before the display of symptoms
- Traveling to an area 21 days prior to an Ebola virus outbreak

Monitoring of Employees That Have Been Exposed to Ebola Virus

Monitoring information of employees that have traveled to an area where there has been an Ebola outbreak or have come in direct contact with an Ebola patient's blood or bodily fluids etc. are as follows:

- Date of potential exposure
- Duration of the exposure
- Mechanism of exposure (via contact with broken skin, blood, bodily fluid, etc.)
- Contact details of physician contacted after exposure
- Consultation provided by the physician
- Monitoring of symptoms during isolation
- Duration of exclusion from work
- Duration of isolation

Training

It is mandatory for nurses, healthcare professionals, doctors, and medical and environmental professionals to be trained and educated about the potential risks of being exposed to the Ebola virus. This is to be provided during work hours and within a safety culture/climate. The routes of transmission as explained prior, along with methods of donning and doffing, protocols for waste management and sanitization are to be disseminated in detail. This also extends to the guidelines regarding what is to be done if exposed to the virus from a PUI or patient diagnosed with the Ebola virus.

Frequency of Training:

The training is to be conducted before the initial assignment of tasks given to nurses, healthcare professionals, doctors, and medical and environmental professionals. This is to be then revised and updated annually or as needed. As new and improved information on the characteristics and containment of the Ebola virus are examined and observed so is the frequency of the training at hand. Personnel that are at a higher risk are to be given more intense training on donning and doffing procedures along with management flows to improve competency and efficiency.

Content that is to be included in the training:

The Ebola prevention and containment content is to incorporate a comprehensive list of elements. They are as follows:

- √ The personnel responsible for the employer's safety and health
- √ Hospital exposure and containment plans
  - Screening and monitoring of incoming patients
  - Patient placement
  - Security and containment measures for patient isolation area
  - Procedures for entry and exit
  - Waste management protocols and placement of materials needed for disposal of waste generated by patients with the Ebola virus
  - Handling of contaminated materials and items
  - Decontamination and sanitization protocols
- √ Protocols to access the medical facilities exposure control plans
- √ Participation methods of employees in plan management
- √ Guidelines for reporting health and safety concerns to management in a prompt manner
- √ List of work tasks that enhance the risk of exposure
- √ Detailed insights into the limitations of personal protective equipment
- √ Process of donning and doffing personal protective equipment

√ How to dispose off personal protective equipment safely

√ Protocols for spillage management

√ How to identify the psychological strain from patient care and personal protective equipment—key markers of identification and way forward

√ Methods of notifying employees or supervisors in case of exposure to the Ebola virus

√ Medical evaluation procedures

Method of pedagogy:

The content related to Ebola virus management, containment, and source control is to be disseminated to nurses, healthcare professionals, doctors, and medical and environmental professionals effectively and efficiently. Interactive sessions where questions can be asked and answered in detail are to be conducted by the medical facility or hospital management. This is to be done by an expert in the field of Ebola exposure control and management to ensure maximum outreach.

In these training sessions, the proper procedures for donning and doffing personal protective equipment and respirators along with patient care and waste management techniques are to be demonstrated in detail.

THE WAY FORWARD

The measures and policies that have been executed, updated, and followed so far have proven to be efficient and effective. With time, however, improvements in technology and research have the potential to develop more robust and dynamic forms of containments.

This extends to vaccination for the Ebola virus as in the cases of polio and HIV among others. While vaccine trials for the Ebola virus may be underway, there is still a long way to go before it becomes accessible and available for the general public. This is largely because the Ebola virus strain is anticipated to mutate, evolve, and transform shortly. All in all, when the provision of the Ebola virus vaccine is to be rolled out the priority is to be given to nurses, healthcare providers, EMS staff, and doctors first. This is because they are at the highest risk of being exposed to the Ebola virus from potentially infected people and confirmed Ebola virus patients.

The challenges going ahead are then to be profound—the ones of ensuring systematic distribution of these vaccines along with vaccine drives. Spreading awareness and knowledge about its benefits and need is going to be a tough journey ahead, especially due to the high level of mistrust and skepticism surrounding vaccines.

Till then, the efforts and sacrifices being made by nurses, healthcare professionals, doctors, and medical and environmental professionals cannot be overlooked. Their constant support and determination to help contain the Ebola virus and help patients with the Ebola virus recover are lauded and praised.

We thank them for their skills, knowledge, patience, willpower, and determination.

GLOSSARY

1. **Active monitoring** – this means that the state or local public health authority assumes responsibility for establishing regular communication with potentially exposed people to assess for the presence of fever, cough, or difficulty breathing. For people with high-risk exposures, CDC recommends this communication occurs at least once each day. The mode of communication can be determined by the state or local public health authority and may include telephone calls or any electronic or internet-based means of communication.

2. **Aerosol Generation Procedures (AGP)** – these procedures extend to procedures that generate aerosols that increase the risk of transmitting respiratory pathogens into the air, thus increasing the chances of air-borne disease outbreaks.

3. **Airborne Infection Isolation Room (AIIR)** – this refers to a formerly, negative pressure isolation room. An AIIR is a single-occupancy patient-care room used to isolate persons with a suspected or confirmed airborne infectious disease. Environmental factors are controlled in AIIRs to minimize the transmission of infectious agents that are usually transmitted from person to person by droplet nuclei associated with coughing or aerosolization of contaminated fluids. AIIRs should provide negative pressure in the room (so that air flows under the door gap into the room); and an airflow rate of 6-12 ACH (6 ACH for existing structures, 12 ACH for new construction or renovation); and direct exhaust of air from the room to the outside of the building or recirculation of air through a HEPA filter before returning to circulation.

4. **Airborne Transmission** – very small particles "droplet nuclei" remain infectious and suspended in the air for extended periods of time. Suspended droplet nuclei undergo desiccation and air currents can disperse droplet nuclei over distances. When inhaled they enter the respiratory tract and can cause infection. This only occurs with infectious agents which are capable of surviving and retaining infectivity for relatively long periods of time. They can be inhaled by susceptible individuals who have not had face-to-face contact or been in the same room with the infected person. Observations of particle dynamics reveal that droplets of 30 μm can also float in the air for periods of time.

5. **Amniotic Fluid** – the fluid that surrounds the growing baby inside the amniotic sac is known as amniotic fluid. It is a clear yellow fluid that facilities the growth of the baby inside the womb.

6. **Antibodies** – also known as immunoglobulin, antibodies are a form of protein that is produced by the immune system. This usually happens in the presence of foreign substances or pathogens that have entered the body.

7. **Antibody-Capture Enzyme-Linked Immunosorbent Assay (ELISA)** – an ELISA is a test that measures the number of antibodies inside the blood. It can also be sued to test proteins and bacterial antigens, hormones, and glycoproteins.

8. **Antigen-Capture Detection Tests** – the Antigen-Capture Detection test is similar to an ELISA that seeks to detect the Ebola Virus pathogen in the blood sample.

9. **Antiseptic Solution** – it is a fluid used to prepare the patient's skin for invasive procedures. It prevents the growth of microorganisms and is mostly isopropyl alcohol or iodine-based.

10. **Anti-Viral Medications** – these drugs are used to target viruses such as influenza, herpes, and hepatitis. They help the body fight off viruses and recover at a faster rate.

11. **Asymptomatic Person** – a person having developed no signs or symptoms of a disease is referred to as being asymptomatic.

12. **Autoclave** – an autoclave is a machine used to decontaminate biological wastes and lab equipment using high temperatures and pressure.

13. **Bacterial Infections** – this is an infection caused when bacteria enter the body and start to multiply. This transmission can occur via being exposed to someone who has a bacterial infection or via contaminated food and water.

14. **Bioaerosols** – an airborne dispersion of particles containing whole or parts of biological entities, such as bacteria, viruses, dust mites, fungal hyphae, or fungal spores. Such aerosols usually consist of a mixture of mono-dispersed and aggregate cells, spores, or viruses, carried by other materials, such as respiratory secretions and/or inert particles. Infectious bioaerosols (i.e., those that contain biological agents capable of causing an infectious disease) can be generated from human sources (e.g., expulsion from the respiratory tract during coughing, sneezing, talking, or singing; during suctioning or wound irrigation), wet environmental sources (e.g. HVAC and cooling tower water with Legionella) or dry sources (e.g., construction dust with spores produced by Aspergillus spp.). Bioaerosols include large respiratory droplets and small droplet nuclei.

15. **Biohazardous** – this term is often used for waste that is highly infectious as it contains potentially transmittable agents that can be hazardous to health.

16. **Biological Containment** – there are several methods used to contain genetically engineered microorganisms. This is known as biological containment and seeks to create biochemical barriers to prevent the hazardous agents from multiplying outside of a facility or laboratory.

17. **Blood Specimen Tests** – these are blood samples collected from the blood vessel by a phlebotomist or medical professionals. The blood sample is then tested to rule out a diagnosis.

18. **Cardiopulmonary Resuscitation** – when a person is unresponsive, cardiopulmonary resuscitation is performed via mouth-to-mouth resuscitation methods. Cardia compressions are also administered to help the circulation of oxygen become reinstated in the body.

19. **Caregivers** – all persons who are not employees of an organization are not paid, and provide or assist in providing healthcare to a patient (e.g., family member, friend) and acquire technical training as needed based on the tasks that must be performed.

20. **Close contact for healthcare exposures is defined as follows:** a) being within approximately 6 feet (2 meters), of a person with 2019-nCoV infection for a prolonged period of time (such as caring for or visiting the patient, or sitting within 6 feet of the patient in a healthcare waiting area or room); or b) having unprotected direct contact with infectious secretions or excretions of the patient (e.g., being coughed on, touching used tissues with a bare hand).

21. **Colonization** – the proliferation of microorganisms on or within body sites without detectable host immune response, cellular damage, or clinical expression. The presence of a microorganism within a host may occur with

varying duration but may become a source of potential transmission. In many instances, colonization and carriage are synonymous.

22. **Contact Transmission** – this can be of two types. Direct: microorganisms are transferred from one infected person to another person without a contaminated intermediate object or person through non-intact skin (cuts, abrasions, dermatitis, chapped skin, scratches, etc.). Indirect transmission is the transfer of infectious agents through a contaminated intermediate object or person (hands of healthcare personnel, patient care devices such as thermometers, stethoscopes, shared toys, inadequately cleaned instruments, soiled garments, or surgical gowns).

23. **Controlled travel** – this involves exclusion from long-distance commercial conveyances (e.g., aircraft, ship, train, bus). For people subject to active monitoring, any long-distance travel should be coordinated with public health authorities to ensure uninterrupted monitoring. Air travel is not allowed by commercial flight but may occur via approved non-commercial air transport.

24. **Diagnosis** – this is the method of identifying, analyzing, and examining a medical condition or disease.

25. **Disinfection** – this refers to the process of destroying or eliminating the growth of microorganisms on a surface. This is done by applying chemical agents or antiseptic solutions.

26. **Disposable Cleaning Materials** – these are items such as aprons, cloths, and other cleaning supplies that are to be discarded as per safety protocols after use.

27. **Donning** – the process of wearing or putting on a clothing item or personal protective equipment.

28. **Doffing** – the process of removing or taking off a clothing item or personal protective equipment.

29. **Droplet Transmission** – a form of contact transmission with the addition of respiratory droplets traveling directly from the respiratory tract of the infected person to susceptible mucosal surfaces of the recipient; eyes/conjunctiva, nasal mucosa, and mouth. Traditionally droplet size is considered > 5 um. Respiratory droplets occur when talking, coughing, sneezing, or during procedures such as tracheal suctioning, endotracheal intubation. Organisms transmitted by the droplet route do not remain infective over long distances and therefore do not require special air handling and ventilation

30. **Drug Therapies** – the administration of medicines or drugs to treat a preventive disease. A combination of various drugs may be used as well. This is referred to as combination therapy.

31. **Ebola Outbreaks** – the spread of the Ebola virus in a new area. It can grow into an epidemic that can affect a large number of people residing in a community or locality over a short period of time.

32. **Electron Microscopy** – this is referred to the process of obtaining high-resolution images of biological and non-biological specimens. It is used for research purposes to study and examine the structure of cells, tissues, and macromolecular complexes.

33. **Emergency Medical Services** – ambulance services that are used during times of emergency are known as Emergency Medical Services. They pro-

vide urgent care and stabilization of the individual in concern until transported to a medical facility.

34. **Employee Health Personnel** – these include nurses, physicians, assistants, medical technicians, or any other authorized personnel acting under the direction of physicians to tend to a patient.

35. **Endotracheal Intubation** – when a patient is unable to breathe properly, an endotracheal tube is placed into the windpipe via the nose or mouth. This is done to protect the airway or sedate an extremely ill patient.

36. **Engineering controls** – this is the removal or isolation of a workplace hazard through technology. AIIRs, a Protective Environment, engineered sharps injury prevention devices, and sharps containers are examples of engineering controls.

37. **Environmental Services Specialists (EVS)** – this refers to personnel that are on the frontline of helping prevent infection. They work in the medical facility and are responsible for maintaining a clean, safe, and healthy environment.

38. **Epidemiologic Risks** – the process of identifying hazards to human health via exposure o intoxicating and infectious agents.

39. **Exposure** – the condition of being subjected to something i.e. infectious agents that can have a harmful effect.

40. **Febrile** – this refers to an illness that has symptoms of fever or high body temperature.

41. **Fetus** – an unborn baby after eight weeks of conception.

42. **Hand hygiene** – this refers to a general term that applies to any one of the following: 1) handwashing with plain (non-antimicrobial) soap and water); 2) antiseptic hand wash (soap containing antiseptic agents and water); 3) antiseptic hand rub (waterless antiseptic product, most often alcohol-based, rubbed on all surfaces of hands); or 4) surgical hand antisepsis (antiseptic handwash or antiseptic hand rub performed preoperatively by surgical personnel to eliminate transient hand flora and reduce resident hand flora).

43. **Healthcare-associated infection (HAI)** – this is an infection that develops in a patient who is cared for in any setting where healthcare is delivered (e.g., acute care hospital, chronic care facility, ambulatory clinic, dialysis center, surgical center, home) and is related to receiving health care (i.e., was not incubating or present at the time healthcare was provided). In ambulatory and home settings, HAI would apply to any infection that is associated with medical or surgical intervention. Since the geographic location of infection acquisition is often uncertain, the preferred term is considered to be healthcare-associated rather than healthcare-acquired.

44. **Healthcare epidemiologist** – a person whose primary training is medical (M.D., D.O.) and/or master or doctorate-level epidemiology who has received advanced training in healthcare epidemiology. Typically, these professionals direct or provide consultation to infection control and prevention program in a hospital, long-term care facility (LTCF), or healthcare delivery system (also see infection control and prevention professional).

45. **Healthcare Personnel** - for the purposes of this document, HCP refers to all paid and unpaid persons serving in healthcare settings who have the potential for direct or indirect exposure to patients or infectious materials, including body substances; contaminated medical supplies, devices, and equipment; contaminated environmental surfaces; or contaminated air. For this document, HCP does not include clinical laboratory personnel.

46. **Healthcare personnel, healthcare workers (HCW)** – all paid and unpaid persons who work in a healthcare setting (e.g. any person who has professional or technical training in a healthcare- related field and provides patient care in a healthcare setting or any person who provides services that support the delivery of healthcare such as dietary, housekeeping, engineering, maintenance personnel).

47. **Hemorrhage** – severe blood loss that can be internal or external.

48. **Heparinized Tubes** – these are tubes used to store blood samples. They are coated on the inside with certain chemicals that help prevent the blood from clotting.

49. **Hepatitis C** – this disease occurs due to the presence of the hepatitis c virus in the boy. It impacts the liver, causing inflammation. The main cause of it is via sharing used needles or coming in contact with the blood from an infected person.

50. **High-efficiency particulate air (HEPA) filter** – this is an air filter that removes >99.97% of particles >0.3μm (the most penetrating particle size) at a specified flow rate of air. HEPA filters may be integrated into the central air handling systems, installed at the point of use above the ceiling of a room, or used as portable units.

51. **Home care** – a wide range of medical, nursing, rehabilitation, hospice, and social services delivered to patients in their place of residence (e.g., private residence, senior living center, assisted living facility). Home health-care services include care provided by home health aides and skilled nurses, respiratory therapists, dieticians, physicians, chaplains, and volunteers; provision of durable medical equipment; home infusion therapy; and physical, speech, and occupational therapy.

52. **Human Immunodeficiency Virus** – this virus attacks the body's immune system, making it a life-threatening condition if left untreated.

53. **Immunocompromised patients** – refers to those patients whose immune mechanisms are deficient because of congenital or acquired immunologic disorders (e.g., human immunodeficiency virus [HIV] infection, congenital immune deficiency syndromes), chronic diseases such as diabetes mellitus, cancer, emphysema, or cardiac failure, ICU care, malnutrition, and immunosuppressive therapy of another disease process [e.g., radiation, cytotoxic chemotherapy, anti-graft rejection medication, corticosteroids, monoclonal antibodies directed against a specific component of the immune system]). The type of infections for which an immunocompromised patient has increased susceptibility is determined by the severity of immunosuppression and the specific component(s) of the immune system that is affected. Patients undergoing allogeneic HSCT and those with chronic graft versus host disease are considered the most vulnerable to HAIs. Immunocompromised states also make it more difficult to diagnose certain infections (e.g., tuberculosis) and are associated with more severe clinical disease states than persons with the same infection and a normal immune system.

54. **Immune Therapies** – this method of curing diseases rests on using certain parts of the patient's immune system to fight off infected cells.

55. **Incineration** – this refers to the process of destroying unwanted material via combustion.

56. **Incubation Period** – the time period during with a person is infected with a disease up until the first signs and symptoms appear.

57. **Infectious** – a contagious substance that can cause disease or illness and be hazardous to health.

58. **Infection** – the transmission of microorganisms into a host after evading or overcoming defense mechanisms, resulting in the organism's proliferation and invasion within host tissue(s). Host responses to infection may include clinical symptoms or maybe subclinical, with manifestations of disease mediated by direct organism's pathogenesis and/or a function of cell-mediated or antibody responses that destroy host tissues.

59. **Infection control and prevention professional (ICP)** – a person whose primary training is in either nursing, medical technology, microbiology, or epidemiology and who has acquired special training in infection control. Responsibilities may include collection, analysis, and feedback of infection data and trends to healthcare providers; consultation on infection risk assessment, prevention and control strategies; performance of education and training activities; implementation of evidence-based infection control practices or those mandated by regulatory and licensing agencies; application of epidemiologic principles to improve patient outcomes; participation in planning renovation and construction projects (e.g., to ensure appropriate containment of construction dust); evaluation of new products

or procedures on patient outcomes; oversight of employee health services related to infection prevention; implementation of preparedness plans; communication within the healthcare setting, with local and state health departments, and with the community at large concerning infection control issues; and participation in research. Certification in infection control (CIC) is available through the Certification Board of Infection Control and Epidemiology.

60. **Infection control and prevention program** – this is a multidisciplinary program that includes a group of activities to ensure that recommended practices for the prevention of healthcare- associated infections are implemented and followed by HCWs, making the healthcare setting safe from infection for patients and healthcare personnel.

61. **The Joint Commission on Accreditation of Healthcare Organizations (JCAHO)** – requires the following five components of an infection control program for accreditation: 1) surveillance: monitoring patients and healthcare personnel for the acquisition of infection and/or colonization; 2) investigation: identification and analysis of infection problems or undesirable trends; 3) prevention: implementation of measures to prevent transmission of infectious agents and to reduce risks for the device- and procedure-related infections; 4) control: evaluation and management of outbreaks; and 5) reporting: provision of information to external agencies as required by state and federal law and regulation. The infection control program staff has the ultimate authority to determine infection control policies for a healthcare organization with the approval of the organization's governing body.

62. **Intrapartum Hemorrhage** – this refers to the severe loss of blood during labor and delivery.

63. **Isolation** – this means the separation of a person or group of people known or reasonably believed to be infected with a communicable disease and potentially infectious from those who are not infected to prevent the spread of the communicable disease. Isolation for public health purposes may be voluntary or compelled by federal, state, or local public health orders.

64. **Malaria** – a disease caused by a parasite that is transmitted into humans via an infected female Anopheles mosquito. Symptoms include high fever, chills, headache, nausea, and vomiting. It can be fatal if left untreated.

65. **Mask** – a term that applies collectively to items used to cover the nose and mouth and includes both procedure masks and surgical masks

66. **Mechanical Ventilators** – a machine that is used to assist a person in breathing while they are having surgery or are unable to breathe on their own.

67. **Medical Evaluations** – medical examinations, tests, and assessments that seek to inspect a person's health status. This includes observing the patient's medical history along with physical examinations conducted by a medical professional.

68. **Medical Procedures** – these include a series of actions and procedures intended to reach a result in the delivery of health care. It may be used to diagnose or treat a pathological or non- pathological condition.

69. **Meningitis** – this is an infection of the fluid (called meninges) surrounding the brain and spinal cord. The viral or bacterial infection causes inflammation and swelling of the membranes that cover the brain or spine.

70. **Monoclonal Antibodies** – these are laboratory-created proteins that act as the immune systems' ability to fight harmful foreign substances such as pathogens. They mimic human antibodies and can restore the normal functioning of the immune system.

71. **Mucous Membranes** – this refers to the thin lining of certain organs and cavities in the body such as the nose, mouth, stomach, and lungs.

72. **N95 Respirator** – a specially designed respiratory protective gear that provides efficient filtration of airborne diseases. It provides a close facial fit and helps prevent airborne transmission. It comes with a filter efficiency of 95%.

73. **Neonates** – a newborn baby or infant that is less than four weeks old.

74. **Negative Pressure** – a relative air pressure difference between two areas. The pressure in a containment room or area that is under negative pressure is lower than adjacent areas which keeps air from flowing out of the containment facility and into adjacent rooms or areas.

75. **Non-Fluid Impermeable** – those elements or materials that do not allow fluids to pass through them.

76. **Non-Invasive Screening Tests** – these are tests that are administered without the use of tools that tear into, break or physically enter the body. Examples of such tests are X-rays, CT scans, MRIs, and ECGs.

77. **Occupational Safety and Health Coordinator** – this refers to a specialist who is responsible for examining the workplace for any internal or external factors that may impact employee safety, health, and performance. They help manage, maintain and execute health and safety programs as well.

78. **Occupational Exposure** – the exposure from work activity or working conditions that are reasonably anticipated to create an elevated risk of contracting any disease caused by ATPs or ATPs-L if protective measures are not in place. In this context elevated means higher than what is considered ordinary for employees having direct contact with the general public outside of the facility. Whether the employee has occupational exposure depends on the tasks, activities, and environment of the employee. Occupational exposure does not exist where a hospital employee works only in an office environment separated from the patient or only works in areas separate from where the risk of ATD transmission, whether from the patient or contaminated items, would be elevated without protective measures.

79. **Open Suctioning of Airways** – this process is also referred to as the endotracheal suctioning technique. It includes disconnecting a patient who is on a ventilator by introducing a suction catheter into the endotracheal tube.

80. **Blood Borne Pathogens** – these are microorganisms in the human blood that are infectious and can cause disease in humans. Some of these diseases include Hepatitis B and HIV.

81. **Powered Air-Purifying Respirators (PAPR)** – a form of respirator worn in places where a high level of protection is needed. It has air-purifying features that remove particles of dust and toxicity from the environment. It uses a blower to force the ambient air through air-purifying elements to the inlet covering.

82. **Pathogens** – these are microorganisms that cause disease when entered into the body. Some of them include bacteria, viruses, and fungi. They are harmful if the immune system is weak and unable to fight it off.

83. **Patient Under Investigation (PUI)** – a person that presents a clinical and epidemiology risk for a certain disease or illness. These signs and risks include 1) elevated fever or body temperature, 2) severe headache, fatigue, muscle pain, vomiting, diarrhea, unexplained hemorrhage, and poses an epidemiological risk factor within the 21 days before the onset of the symptoms.

84. **Perinatal Death** – this refers to the early neonatal death of an infant or a stillbirth.

85. **Perinatal Mortality Rates** – the incidence of perinatal deaths divided by total births.

86. **Personal protective equipment (PPE)** – a variety of barriers used alone or in combination to protect mucous membranes, skin, and clothing from contact with infectious agents. PPE includes gloves, masks, respirators, goggles, face shields, and gowns.

87. **Phlebotomy** – the process of drawing blood from the vein via a needle. The blood may then be used for laboratory testing or to treat blood disorders.

88. **Pneumatic Tube System** – a system designed to safely and efficiently transport physical objects such as blood samples, medications, or injections. They help save time and keep infectious and hazardous elements from coming in contact with the human body.

89. **Procedure Mask** – this refers to a covering for the nose and mouth that is intended for use in general patient care situations. These masks generally attach to the face with ear loops rather than ties or elastic. Unlike surgical masks, procedure masks are not regulated by the Food and Drug Administration.

90. **Protective Environment** – a specialized patient-care area, usually in a hospital, that has a positive airflow relative to the corridor (i.e., air flows from the room to the outside adjacent space). The 64 combination of high-efficiency particulate air (HEPA) filtration, high numbers (>12) of air changes per hour (ACH), and minimal leakage of air into the room creates an environment that can safely accommodate patients with a severely compromised immune system (e.g., those who have received allogeneic hemopoietin stem-cell transplant [HSCT]) and decrease the risk of exposure to spores produced by environmental fungi. Other components include the use of scrubbable surfaces instead of materials such as upholstery or carpeting, cleaning to prevent dust accumulation, and prohibition of fresh flowers or potted plants.

91. **Public health orders** – these are legally enforceable directives issued under the authority of a relevant federal, state or local entity that, when applied to a person or group, may place restrictions on the activities undertaken by that person or group, potentially including movement restrictions or a requirement for monitoring by a public health authority, for the purposes of protecting the public's health. Federal, state, or local public health orders may be issued to enforce isolation, quarantine, or conditional release.

92. **Quarantine** – in general quarantine means the separation of a person or group of people reasonably believed to have been exposed to a communicable disease but not yet symptomatic, from others who have not been so exposed, to prevent the possible spread of the communicable disease.

93. **Radiology Technicians** – these are specialists who are responsible for performing imaging procedures such as CT scans, X-rays, and MRI scans.

94. **Recovery** – the process of returning to a healthy state both mentally and physically.

95. **Respirator** – a personal protective device worn by healthcare personnel to protect them from inhalation exposure to airborne infectious agents that are < 5 µm in size. These include infectious droplet nuclei from patients with M. tuberculosis, variola virus [smallpox], SARS-CoV), and dust particles that contain infectious particles, such as spores of environmental fungi (e.g., Aspergillus sp.). The CDC's National Institute for Occupational Safety and Health (NIOSH) certifies respirators used in healthcare settings. The N95 disposable particulate, air-purifying, a respirator is the type used most commonly by healthcare personnel. Other respirators used include N-99 and N-100 particulate respirators, powered air-purifying respirators (PAPRS) with high-efficiency filters; and non-powered full-facepiece elastomeric negative pressure respirators. Respirators must be used in conjunction with a complete Respiratory Protection Program, as required by the Occupational Safety and Health Administration (OSHA), that includes fit testing, training, proper selection of respirators, medical clearance, and respirator maintenance.

96. **Respiratory Hygiene/ Cough Etiquette** – a combination of measures designed to minimize the transmission of respiratory pathogens via droplet or airborne routes in healthcare settings. The components of Respiratory Hygiene/Cough Etiquette are 1) covering the mouth and nose during coughing and sneezing, 2) using tissues to contain respiratory secretions with prompt disposal into a no-touch receptacle, 3) offering a surgical mask to persons who are coughing to decrease contamination of the surrounding environment, and 4) turning the head away from others and maintaining spatial separation, ideally >3 feet, when coughing. These measures are

targeted to all patients with symptoms of respiratory infection and their accompanying family members or friends beginning at the point of the initial encounter with a healthcare setting (e.g., reception/triage in emergency departments, ambulatory clinics, healthcare provider offices).

97. **Reverse Transcriptase Polymerase Chain Reaction (RT-PCR)** – this is a test used to detect the genetic makeup of a specific organism such as a virus that may be present inside the human body.

98. **Safety culture/climate** – the shared perceptions of workers and management regarding the expectations of safety in the work environment. A hospital safety climate includes the following six organizational components: 1) senior management support for safety programs; 2) absence of workplace barriers to safe work practices; 3) cleanliness and orderliness of the worksite; 4) minimal conflict and good communication among staff members; 5) frequent safety-related feedback/training by supervisors; and 6) availability of PPE and engineering controls.

99. **Self-monitoring** – this means people should monitor themselves for fever by taking their temperatures twice a day and remaining alert for cough or difficulty breathing. Anyone on self- monitoring should be provided a plan for whom to contact if they develop fever, cough, or difficulty breathing during the self-monitoring period to determine whether the medical evaluation is needed.

100. **Self-observation** – this means people should remain alert for subjective fever, cough, or difficulty breathing. If they feel feverish or develop cough or difficulty breathing during the self-observation period, they should take their temperature, limit contact with others, and seek.

101. **Self-monitoring with delegated supervision** – this means, for certain occupational groups (e.g., some healthcare or laboratory personnel, airline crew members), self-monitoring with oversight by the appropriate occupational health or infection control program in coordination with the health department of jurisdiction. The occupational health or infection control personnel for the employing organization should establish points of contact between the organization, the self-monitoring personnel, and the local or state health departments with jurisdiction for the location where self-monitoring personnel will be during the self-monitoring period. This communication should result in agreement on a plan for medical evaluation of personnel who develop fever, cough, or difficulty breathing during the self-monitoring period. The plan should include instructions for notifying occupational health and the local public health authority, and transportation arrangements to a pre-designated hospital, if medically necessary, with advance notice if fever, cough, or difficulty breathing occur. The supervising organization should remain in contact with personnel through the self-monitoring period to oversee self-monitoring activities.

102. **Self-monitoring with public health supervision** – this means public health authorities assume the responsibility for oversight of self-monitoring for certain groups of people. CDC recommends that health departments establish initial communication with these people, provide a plan for self-monitoring and clear instructions for notifying the health department before the person seeks health care if they develop fever, cough, or difficulty breathing, and as resources allow, check-in intermittently with these people over the course of the self-monitoring period. If travelers for whom public health supervision is recommended are identified at a US port of entry, CDC will notify state and territorial health departments with jurisdiction for the travelers' final destinations.

103. **Serologic Testing** – this procedure involves identifying antibodies in the blood.

104. **Serum Neutralization Test** – this test measures the ability of a patient's antibodies to neutralize and protect the cells from infection.

105. **Social distancing** – remaining out of congregate settings, avoiding local public transportation (e.g., bus, subway, taxi, rideshare), and maintaining distance (approximately 6 feet or 2 meters) from others. If social distancing is recommended, presence in congregate settings or use of local public transportation should only occur with the approval of local or state health authorities.

106. **Source Control** – this is the process of containing an infectious agent either at the portal of exit from the body or within a confined space. The term is applied most frequently to the containment of infectious agents transmitted by the respiratory route but could apply to other routes of transmission, (e.g., a draining wound, vesicular or bullous skin lesions). Respiratory Hygiene/Cough Etiquette that encourages individuals to "cover your cough" and/or wear a mask is a source control measure. The use of enclosing devices for local exhaust ventilation (e.g., booths for sputum induction or administration of aerosolized medication) is another example of source control.

107. **Standard Precautions** – a group of infection prevention practices that apply to all patients, regardless of suspected or confirmed diagnosis or presumed infection status. Standard Precautions is a combination and expansion of Universal Precautions 780 and Body Substance Isolation 1102. Standard Precautions is based on the principle that all blood, body fluids, secretions, excretions except sweat, non-intact skin, and mucous mem-

branes may contain transmissible infectious agents. Standard Precautions include hand hygiene, and depending on the anticipated exposure, use of gloves, gown, mask, eye protection, or face shield. Also, equipment or items in the patient environment likely to have been contaminated with infectious fluids must be handled in a manner to prevent transmission of infectious agents, (e.g. wear gloves for handling, contain heavily soiled equipment, properly clean and disinfect or sterilize reusable equipment before use on another patient).

108. **Symptoms** – a noticeable and experienced sign of an illness or disease.

109. **Surgical mask** – this is a device worn over the mouth and nose by operating room personnel during surgical procedures to protect both surgical patients and operating room personnel from the transfer of microorganisms and body fluids. Surgical masks also are used to protect healthcare personnel from contact with large infectious droplets (>5 μm in size). According to draft guidance issued by the Food and Drug Administration on May 15, 2003, surgical masks are evaluated using standardized testing procedures for fluid resistance, bacterial filtration efficiency, differential pressure (air exchange), and flammability in order to mitigate the risks to health associated with the use of surgical masks. These specifications apply to any masks that are labeled surgical, laser, isolation, or dental or medical procedure. Surgical masks do not protect against inhalation of small particles or droplet nuclei and should not be confused with particulate respirators that are recommended for protection against selected airborne infectious agents, (e.g., Mycobacterium tuberculosis).

110. **Transplacental Viral Passage** – the transmission of a virus via the placenta, usually from the mother to the unborn baby.

111. **Transmission** – the spread of an infectious agent from one person to another.

112. **Treatment** – the process of medical care to help recover from a disease. This can include several procedures such as using medications, surgery, radiation, physiotherapy, etc.

113. **Typhoid** – a bacterial infection that is caused by the bacteria Salmonella typhi. It is transmitted via contaminated food and water and results in high fever, nausea, and weakness that can be fatal if left untreated.

114. **Umbilical Cord** – a tube that connects the baby to the mother during pregnancy. It helps carry nutrients and oxygen from the placenta to the baby.

115. **Vaccine** – a biological substance that is designed to protect the human body from bacterial or viral infections. It helps enhance the body's natural defenses to build immunity to fight off the pathogen if it enters the body.

116. **Virus** - a pathogen that is infectious and can only multiply inside living cells, killing the host cell in the process.

117. **Virus Isolation** – the process of isolating and identifying virus specimens.

118. **Waste Management** – the processes and procedures involved in managing unwanted materials. It starts from the generation of the waste and extends up till the final disposal.

119. **Zoonotic Disease** – an infectious disease that can be transmitted between human and animal species.

REFERENCES

2014-2016 Ebola Outbreak in West Africa. (n.d.). Retrieved from CDC: https://www.cdc.gov/vhf/ebola/history/2014-2016-outbreak/index.html?CDC_AA_refVal=https%3A%2F%2Fwww.cdc.gov%2Fvhf%2Febola%2Foutbreaks%2F2014-west-africa%2Findex.html

Advancing the Safe Transportation of Energy and Hazardous Materials. (n.d.). Retrieved from Pipeline and Hazardous Materials Safety Administration: https://www.phmsa.dot.gov/

Care of a Neonate Born to a Mother who is Confirmed to have Ebola, is a Person under Investigation, or has been Exposed to Ebola. (n.d.). Retrieved from CDC: https://www.cdc.gov/vhf/ebola/clinicians/evd/neonatal-care.html

CDC Tightened Guidance for U.S. Healthcare Workers on Personal Protective Equipment for Ebola. (n.d.). Retrieved from Centers for Disease Control and Prevention: https://www.cdc.gov/media/releases/2014/fs1020-ebola-personal-protective-equipment.html

Centers for Diesease Control and Prevention . (n.d.). Retrieved from Guidance on Personal Protective Equipment (PPE) To Be Used By Healthcare Workers during Management of Patients with Confirmed Ebola or Persons under Investigation (PUIs): personal protective equipment (PPE)(http://www.cdc.gov/vhf/ebola/hcp/procedures-for-ppe.html) andenvironmentalinfectioncontrol(http://www.cdc.gov/vhf/ebola/hcp/environmental-infection-control-in-hospitals.html)

Ebola Virus Disease . (n.d.). Retrieved from Centers for Disease Control and

Prevention: http://www.cdc.gov/vhf/ebola/index.html

Ebola Virus Disease Distribution Map: Cases of Ebola Virus Disease in Africa Since 1976. (n.d.). Retrieved from Centers for Disease Control and Prevention: Source: https://www.cdc.gov/vhf/ebola/history/distribution-map.html

Ebola-Associated Waste Management. (n.d.). Retrieved from Centers for Disease Control and Prevention:
https://www.cdc.gov/vhf/ebola/clinicians/cleaning/waste-management.html

For Clinicians. (n.d.). Retrieved from Centers for Disease Control and Prevention: https://www.cdc.gov/vhf/ebola/clinicians/index.html

Guidance for Screening and Caring for Pregnant Women with Ebola Virus Disease for Healthcare Providers in U.S. Hospitals. (n.d.). Retrieved from CDC:
https://www.cdc.gov/vhf/ebola/clinicians/evd/pregnant-women.html

Guidance on Personal Protective Equipment (PPE) To Be Used By Healthcare Workers. (n.d.). Retrieved from Centers for Disease Control and Prevention:
http://www.cdc.gov/vhf/ebola/hcp/procedures-for-ppe.html

Identify, Isolate, Inform: Emergency Department Evaluation and Management for Patients Under Investigation (PUIs) for Ebola Virus Disease (EVD). (n.d.). Retrieved from Centers for Disease Control and Prevention:
http://www.cdc.gov/vhf/ebola/hcp/ed-management-patients-possible-ebola.html

Infection Prevention and Control Recommendations for Hospitalized Patients Under Investigation (PUIs) for Ebola Virus Disease (EVD). (n.d.). Retrieved from CDC: https://www.cdc.gov/vhf/ebola/clinicians/evd/infection-control.html

Infection Prevention and Control Recommendations for Hospitalized Patients Under Investigation (PUIs) for Ebola Virus Disease (EVD) in U.S. Hospitals. (n.d.). Retrieved from CDC: https://www.cdc.gov/vhf/ebola/clinicians/evd/infection-control.html

Information on the Survivability of the Ebola Virus in Medical Waste. (n.d.). Retrieved from Centers for Disease Control and Prevention: http://www.cdc.gov/vhf/ebola/hcp/survivability-ebola-medical-waste.html

Interim Guidance for Emergency Medical Services (EMS) Systems and 9-1-1 Emergency Communications Centers/Public Safety Answering Points (ECC/PSAPs) for Management of Patients Under Investigation (PUIs) for Ebola Virus Disease (EVD) in the United States. (n.d.). Retrieved from CDC: https://www.cdc.gov/vhf/ebola/clinicians/emergency-services/ems-systems.html

Interim Guidance for Environmental Infection Control in Hospitals for Ebola Virus. (n.d.). Retrieved from Centers for Disease Control and Prevention: http://www.cdc.gov/vhf/ebola/hcp/environmental-infection-control-in-hospitals.html

Interim Guidance for Environmental Infection Control in Hospitals for Ebola Virus. (n.d.). Retrieved from Centers for Disease Control and Prevention: http://www.cdc.gov/vhf/ebola/hcp/environmental-infection-control-in-hospitals.html

Interim Guidance for Specimen Collection, Transport, Testing, and Submission for Patients with Suspected Infection with Ebola Virus Disease. (n.d.). Retrieved from CDC: http://www.cdc.gov/vhf/ebola/pdf/ebola-lab-guidance.pdf

(2019). KAISER PERMANENTE - Ebola Exposure Control Plan. Retrieved from Ebola Exposure Control Plan

Packaging and Shipping Clinical Specimens Diagram. (n.d.). Retrieved from CDC: https://www.cdc.gov/vhf/ebola/laboratory-personnel/shipping-specimens.html

Q&A's about the Transport of Pediatric Patients (< 18 years of age) Under Investigation or with Confirmed Ebola. (n.d.). Retrieved from CDC: https://www.cdc.gov/vhf/ebola/clinicians/emergency-services/transporting-pediatric-patients.html

RESPIRATORS. (n.d.). Retrieved from CDC: https://www.cdc.gov/niosh/topics/respirators/

Screening Patients. (n.d.). Retrieved from CDC: https://www.cdc.gov/vhf/ebola/clinicians/evaluating-patients/index.html?CDC_AA_refVal=https%3A%2F%2Fwww.cdc.gov%2Fvhf%2Febola%2Fclinicians%2Fevaluating-patients%2Fcase-definition.html

Signs and Symptoms. (n.d.). Retrieved from Centers for Disease Control and Prevention: http://www.cdc.gov/vhf/ebola/symptoms/index.html

Transmission. (n.d.). Retrieved from Centers for Disease Control and Prevention: http://www.cdc.gov/vhf/ebola/transmission/human-transmission.html

U.S. DOT Guidance for Transporting Ebola Contaminated Items, a Category A Infectious Substance FAQs. (n.d.). Retrieved from CDC: http://phmsa.dot.gov/hazmat/transporting-infectious-substances/packaging-of-ebola-contaminated-waste/faq

U.S. EPA Disinfectants for Use Against the Ebola Virus. (n.d.). Retrieved from CDC: http://www.epa.gov/oppad001/list-l-ebola-virus.html

For 20 Continuing Education units,

go to www.Nursing-CEs.com and use Code DOR22 for your free CE units.